To my mother Marijke, who has been showing me for more than half a century that you can do anything if you want and that you should not let anything or anyone stop you from doing so.

"In these days when science is clearly in the saddle and when our knowledge of disease is advancing at a breathless pace, we are apt to forget that not all can ride and that he also serves who waits and who applies what the horseman discovers."

(Harvey Cushing)

The PPID Book

Remco Sikkel

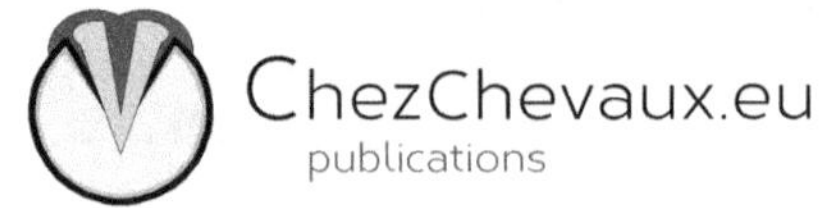

Original title: Het PPID-boek

Cover images: Nikkie de Kerf (horse),
Michael Frank, Royal Veterinary College, London (brains)

Photo credits: see page 170

understandinglaminitis.com
fb.me/understandinglaminitis

By the same author:
• The Laminitis answer book : over 200 questions answered
  (ISBN 978-94-93034-10-5)
• Laminitis : understanding, cure, prevention
  (ISBN 978-94-93034-09-9)

This book is not intended to replace the professional advice of a veterinarian, hoof care
provider, equine nutritionist or any other horse health care specialist. It merely provides
an overview of the current theories, diagnostic and treatment methods relating to PPID
and its complications. The reader should always consult a veterinarian in matters relating
to their horse's health and, in particular, in relation to clinical signs or complications of PPID
or laminitis requiring diagnosis or medical attention. Neither the author, nor the publisher,
nor the photographers can be held liable for any resulting damage from the application of
the information contained in this book.

TABLE OF CONTENTS

SIDEBARS

HOW TO READ THIS BOOK

PPID is a very complex subject. There is a lot to say about it. So, a line has to be drawn somewhere to avoid overwhelming you, the reader of this book, with details. In this book, that has been done in a particular way.

‖ Read everything if you want to know all the ins and outs, but if that is too much for you in one sitting, you can skip the in-depth paragraphs to get a general overview. You will recognise them by a double vertical line to the left of the text, as in the text you are reading now. When you've finished reading the book and flip through the pages later, your curiosity may win out after all.

A summary is provided at the end of each chapter.

On page 171 you will find a glossary.

> GLOSSARY TERM
> The first time a glossary term appears in the text, it looks like this.

Some bits of text are given special attention in the form of a 'nota bene'.

AND THEN THERE ARE SIDEBARS
They provide background information to give you more context.

INTRODUCTION

*Before delving into all aspects of PPID, this chapter provides a brief overview
of the disease, its prevalence, and which equines are affected.*

PPID

Pituitary Pars Intermedia Dysfunction, or PPID for short, is a slowly developing and incurable impairment of part of the nervous system. Whilst mainly impacting older horses it can also affect younger ones, as well as donkeys, mules, and hinnies. Since horses are living with us for an ever increasing lifespan, it becomes increasingly important that we understand what PPID is and learn how to deal with it.

Simply put, nerves travel from the hypothalamus, a part of the brain, to the pituitary gland, a hormone-producing gland at the brain's base. These nerves produce the hormone dopamine, which is meant to inhibit part of the pituitary gland's production of other important hormones. In PPID, these nerves are damaged and gradually deteriorate. As a result, there's less dopamine available to inhibit the pituitary gland. With the pituitary gland's hormone production losing its proper regulation, things can go haywire. This causes a slew of issues in the horse's body.

The pituitary gland can eventually swell and put pressure on surrounding nerve and brain tissue. This, in turn, causes additional issues for the horse.

HORMONAL DISORDER

The hormonal disorder caused by PPID is known to all veterinarians nowadays. However, there are numerous aspects of how the disease initiates and advances that remain unclear. We're still in the process of learning and discovering new things about diagnosis, treatment and prevention.

The overproduced pituitary hormones affect many different bodily functions. As a result, different horses may show a different clinical presentation.

The clinical presentation encompasses all the clinical signs of disease. A clinical sign is a disease characteristic that can be objectively determined.

The disease progression rate can also differ significantly between horses. Nevertheless, PPID typically starts slowly and can easily go unnoticed in its early stages, making it easy to overlook.

EPIDEMIOLOGY

Epidemiology is concerned, among other things, with how frequently and in whom a disease occurs, as well as what factors contribute to this.

HOW FREQUENTLY

Despite the increase in PPID diagnoses and treatments over the past two decades, there is no evidence to suggest that PPID is becoming more prevalent. It is just that horses with PPID are less likely to stay under the radar. This is because the clinical manifestations of PPID are no longer considered as a natural part of the ageing process.

Diagnostics have also advanced significantly in recent years, and testing is now performed on a more regular basis. When drawing blood to test for insulin dysregulation, it is not uncommon for the vet to also screen for PPID. Furthermore, thanks to the scientific community's increased focus on PPID, a broader audience now has access to new discoveries and insights.

As a result, horse owners have a better understanding of the disease and are more likely to raise the alarm if they suspect their horse has PPID.

Nonetheless, horse owners' level of knowledge could be better. Studies indicate that they often identify PPID too late or fail to recognise clear clinical signs at all [32, 41] *. As a result, horse owners can sometimes react very late, which, in the case of progressive and irreversible disease, would preferably be avoided.

Your hoof care provider, equine dentist, nutritionist, or any other professional who works with your horse is also more likely to alert you to PPID-related issues. They now have greater access to new scientific knowledge about the disease as well.

IN WHOM

Although PPID has been identified in a horse as young as five years old, advanced age remains the most important predictor. Simply put, the older the horse, the more likely it is to develop PPID. This is demonstrated by the fact that veterinarians diagnose PPID in older horses more frequently than in young horses. This conclusion is consistent with the clinical signs observed by horse owners.

---

*   You will find the bibliography on page 157

PPID is diagnosed in just over 20% of horses over the age of 15, and almost 3% of all domestic equines. One out of every three horses over 30 years old has the condition [102].

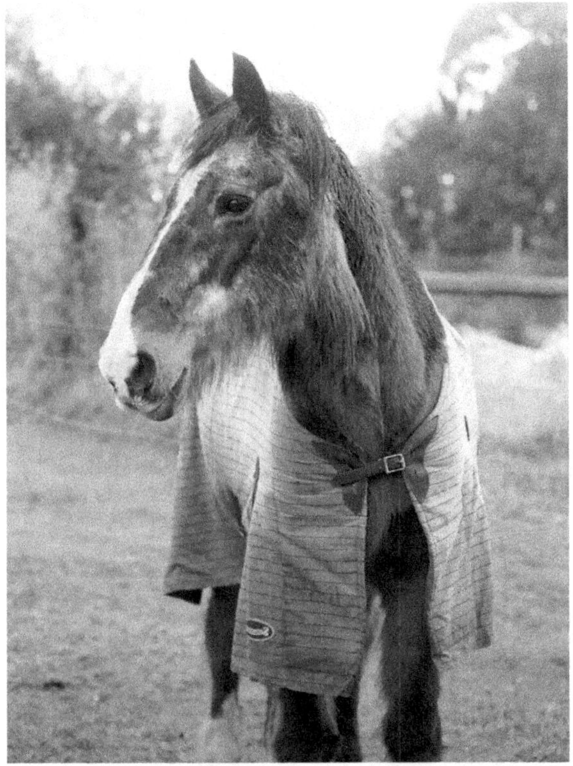

The older the horse, the higher the risk of PPID

(photo: Pat Whelen)

A 2013 study found that horses aged 15 and above face an 18% increased risk of PPID for every year of life [214].

In a comprehensive 2016 study involving horses of all ages, the average age at diagnosis of PPID was 21 years [215].

After diagnosis, their average life expectancy was close to ten years, which is a significant improvement compared to the four and a half years expectancy recorded in horses with PPID from a previous 2012 study [51].

Ponies with a healthy weight undergoing pergolide treatment show the most favourable prognosis [122].

Conservative estimates suggest that PPID is about ten to fifteen times more common than Parkinson's disease in humans, a condition that shares some similarities with PPID [6].

Some studies suggest a higher PPID prevalence in specific pony breeds compared to horses. However, due to the overrepresentation of ponies in these studies, it is not possible to definitively conclude that breed is a risk factor [102].

The only study conducted so far that specifically investigated 'pony' as a risk factor, found no difference in the chances of development of PPID between horses and ponies [214].

Ponies are more prone to developing coat issues associated with PPID than horses [32, 212]. The same applies for laminitis. This may lead veterinarians and horse owners to perceive ponies as more susceptible to PPID than horses.

Some researchers believe that mares face a higher risk of PPID compared to geldings and stallions [96, 145], while others hold the opposite view [126, 247]. To avoid confusion, we can set aside these conflicting findings and assume that gender does not predict PPID.

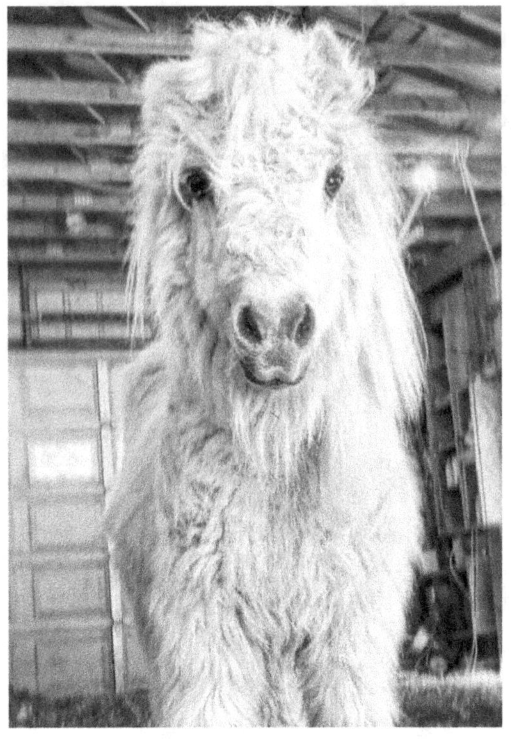

Coat changes in a pony with PPID
(photo: Barabara Trotman)

SUMMARY

PPID is a slowly progressive and irreversible impairment of the dopamine-producing nerves running from the hypothalamus to the pituitary gland. As a result, there is a lack of dopamine, leading to insufficient inhibition of hormone production in part of the pituitary gland. This initiates a series of hormonal imbalances, resulting in a whole range of health issues. Over time, the swelling of the pituitary gland can exert pressure on surrounding brain tissue.

The older the horse, the more likely it is to develop PPID. It has not been proven that the disease is more common in certain breeds or that gender has an influence.

ANATOMY AND PHYSIOLOGY

PPID is a complex disease that manifests itself in different areas of the body. It starts with nerves in the brain, endocrine glands and the hormones they produce, extending to muscles, tendons, bones, fatty tissue, hooves, sweat glands, hair follicles, and many more organs and tissues. To understand PPID, we will start by examining the hypothalamus, pituitary and adrenal glands in this chapter. We will explore the anatomy and physiology of other affected tissues later in the book.

HYPOTHALAMUS

The hypothalamus, an endocrine gland, is a part of the brain; the inter-brain (or diencephalon) to be precise. Blood vessels and nerve cells connect the hypothalamus to the adjacent pituitary gland. The nerve cells release hormones, allowing the hypothalamus to regulate specific functions of the pituitary gland.

DOPAMINE

One of these hormones is dopamine, a neurotransmitter that regulates the intermediate lobe (or middle lobe) of the pituitary gland in the production of hormones known as melanocortins. Dopamine acts as an inhibitor, slowing down their production.

NEUROTRANSMITTER
Endogenous chemical responsible for transmitting nerve signals.

Dopamine also acts on the anterior lobe (or frontal lobe) of the pituitary gland. Some clinical signs of PPID are linked to this. While dopamine serves various functions in the body, our focus in this book will be on its inhibitory effect on the pituitary gland.

TRH

The intermediate lobe is stimulated by the hypothalamus with the hormone TRH (thyrotropin-releasing hormone). Simply put, TRH is the accelerator and dopamine is the brake in melanocortin production.

Whilst the exact pathway of how TRH reaches the nerve cells is still unclear, it is either via nerves, as is the case in amphibians, or through the bloodstream.

PITUITARY GLAND

The pituitary gland, or pituitary for short, is a hormone-producing gland located at the base of the brain. It is about the size of a large cocoa bean (2 x 2 x 1 cm / 0.8 x 0.8 x 0.4 inches) and weighs around three grams (0.1 oz). This gland lies within a cavity at the base of the skull, known as the Turkish saddle.

The pituitary gland secretes stimulating hormones that control the activity of endocrine glands in other parts of the body.

The pituitary gland is divided into three parts or lobes: the anterior (or frontal) lobe, the intermediate (or middle) lobe, and the posterior (or back) lobe. The Latin names are *pars anterior*, *pars intermedia* and *pars posterior*, respectively.

The anterior and intermediate lobes together are referred to as the adeno-hypophysis (hypophysis is another name for the pituitary gland). The anterior lobe merges into the tubular lobe (*pars tuberalis*). To keep it simple, we consider this lobe to be part of the anterior lobe.

The intermediate lobe consists of melanotropes, which are hormone-producing cells directly controlled by the dopamine-producing nerves of the hypothalamus.

Dopamine binds to so-called D2 receptors on the melanotropes, inhibiting the activity of these cells.

A receptor is a part of a cell that has specialised to perceive (hormonal) stimuli, and to trigger a reaction in response to these stimuli.

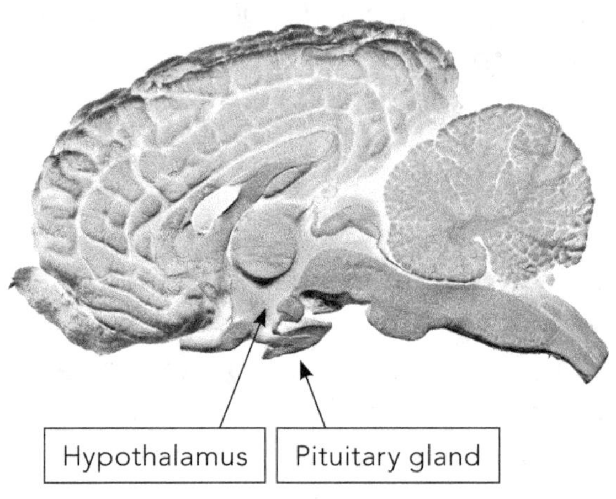

Cross-section of the brain

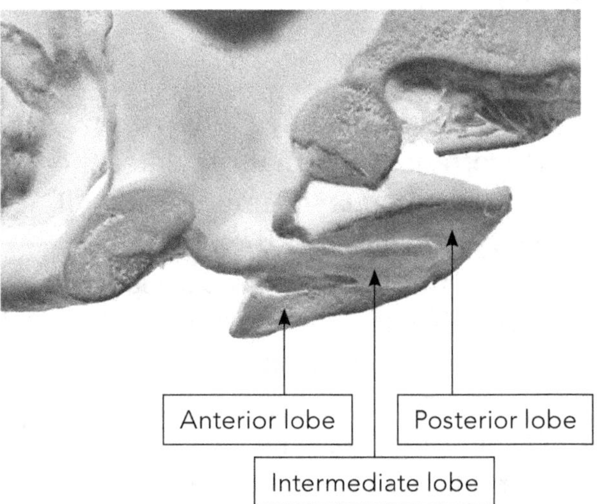

Detailed section of brain: pituitary gland
(*photo: Michael Frank, Royal Veterinary College*)

POMC AND MELANOCORTINS

Melanotropes produce the protein POMC (pro-opiomelanocortin). POMC is a so-called pro-hormone. Special enzymes (pro-hormone convertases PC1 and PC2) cleave it into different hormones in several steps. These resulting hormones are collectively referred to as melanocortins. Dopamine inhibits both the production and the cleavage of POMC.

The melanocortins we will be discussing in this book are:
- ACTH
  - Alpha-MSH
  - CLIP
- Beta-endorphin

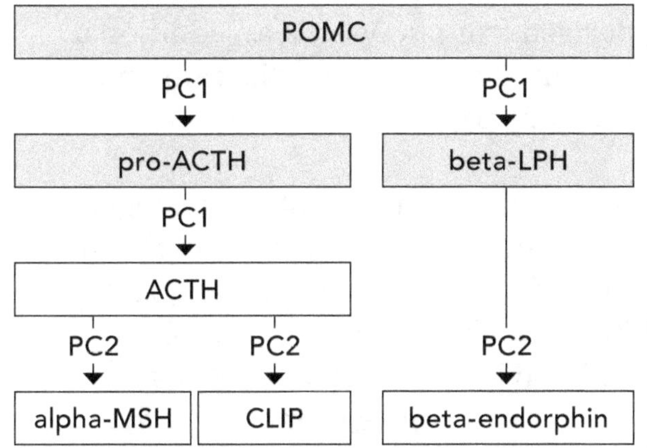

A simplified representation of melanocortin production

N.B. the pro-hormones pro-ACTH and beta-LPH are not discussed further in this book

> **PRO-HORMONE**
> A precursor of a hormone. It usually has little or no hormonal effect itself.

POMC is also produced by nerve cells in the anterior lobe (corticotropes), which is converted into ACTH as well. This ACTH is not cleaved into alpha-MSH or CLIP. This is a process unique to the intermediate lobe.

ACTH

ACTH, short for adrenocorticotropic hormone, is a hormone and neurotransmitter that stimulates the production of corticosteroids, such as cortisol, in the adrenal cortex.

> **CORTICOSTEROIDS**
> Hormones produced by the adrenal cortex, which can be categorised into glucocorticoids and mineralocorticoids. In the context of PPID, the primary involvement is with glucocorticoids.

Since almost all ACTH from the intermediate lobe is converted to alpha-MSH and CLIP, the anterior lobe of the pituitary gland is the primary source of ACTH in healthy horses. Approximately 98% of the ACTH circulating in their blood originates in the anterior lobe [218].

ALPHA-MSH

Alpha-MSH, which stands for alpha-melanocyte-stimulating hormone, is a cleaving product of ACTH. It is main hormonal output of the pituitary intermediate lobe [119].

Alpha-MSH plays a role in metabolism and has effects such as countering the appetite-suppressing actions of the hormone leptin, which we will discuss later. It is likely that the increased production of alpha-MSH as days get shorter serves as a survival strategy to store fat for the winter months when feed may become scarce [231]. In the months leading up to winter, we see that nearly all horses put on weight.

> **METABOLISM**
> The totality of physical and chemical processes that take place within living cells for the maintenance, breakdown and construction of tissue as well as for energy production.

Although alpha-MSH has an anti-inflammatory effect, which is 23 times stronger than paracetamol [93], it may also cause increased pain sensitivity.

Alpha-MSH can have up to a sixfold enhancement on the biological activity of ACTH [53]. Therefore, in PPID-affected horses, the modest amount of ACTH released into the circulation from the intermediate lobe can result in a rather substantial effect [228].

CLIP

This acronym stands for corticotropin-like intermediate lobe peptide. It is a hormone that is also cleaved from ACTH. Its precise mechanism of action is still unknown. In rats, it stimulates the pancreas to produce insulin [63, 106]. Whether this is also the case in horses remains uncertain. Insulin will be discussed in detail later in this book.

BETA-ENDORPHIN

The hormone beta-endorphin, although a cleaving product of POMC, is not produced from ACTH. It is rather derived from POMC via an additional intermediate step (see diagram on the previous page).

Beta-endorphin is a potent, endogenous opium-like substance that has analgesic and anti-inflammatory properties. In PPID-afflicted horses, the opioid action of beta-endorphin seems to be significantly more pronounced than in healthy horses [105].

Like alpha-MSH, beta-endorphin can potentiate the effect of ACTH sixfold [15].

ADRENAL GLANDS

The adrenal glands, also known as suprarenal glands, are small hormone glands situated atop the kidneys. They release various hormones, called adrenal hormones. In the context of PPID, we mainly look at cortisol.

The adrenal hormones are further divided into adrenal cortex hormones and adrenal medullary hormones, depending on which part of the adrenal glands they're produced in.

Cortisol has several functions in the body, some of which we will discuss in this book. One important function, which we will mention here, is the inhibitory effect that cortisol has on the hormone release of the anterior lobe of the pituitary gland. Cortisol has no such effect on the intermediate lobe. The latter is only inhibited by dopamine from the hypothalamus.

We will also briefly touch on androgens (male sex hormones) and adrenaline as adrenal hormones.

SUMMARY

The hypothalamus is a hormone gland in the brain. Nerve cells of the hypothalamus secrete dopamine. This hormone inhibits the action of the intermediate lobe of the pituitary gland.

The pituitary gland is also a hormone gland. It produces ACTH, alpha-MSH, CLIP and beta-endorphin. These are collectively known as melanocortins. A healthy horse's melanocortin production is kept in check by dopamine.

Cortisol and other adrenal hormones are produced by the adrenal glands. One of the functions of cortisol is to inhibit the anterior lobe of the pituitary gland.

DESCRIPTION

The terms PPID, Cushing's disease, and Cushing's syndrome are often confused or used interchangeably. However, these are three distinct issues. We will briefly discuss Cushing's disease and syndrome before delving into PPID.

CUSHING'S DISEASE

American neurosurgeon Harvey Williams Cushing first identified this condition in a human in 1912. Cushing's disease is characterised by a benign glandular tissue tumour, called adenoma, which forms in the anterior lobe of the pituitary gland. As a result, this tissue secretes too much ACTH. This causes overactivity and enlargement of the adrenal glands, resulting in excessive cortisol production.

The clinical signs of Cushing's disease are primarily attributed to the effect of chronically elevated cortisol levels, a condition known as hypercortisolaemia. Unlike in dogs and humans, this disease is virtually non-existent in horses.

CUSHING'S SYNDROME

Fuller Albright, an American endocrinologist, first defined Cushing's syndrome in 1943. It is a collective term for all disorders induced by a chronic excess of cortisol in the blood. The latter could be due to Cushing's disease – which, as mentioned, is extremely unlikely in horses –, but long-term use of synthetic corticosteroids also promotes hypercortisolaemia.

Though uncommon, a malignant tumour, an adenoma, or any other condition of the adrenal glands could be the cause [97].

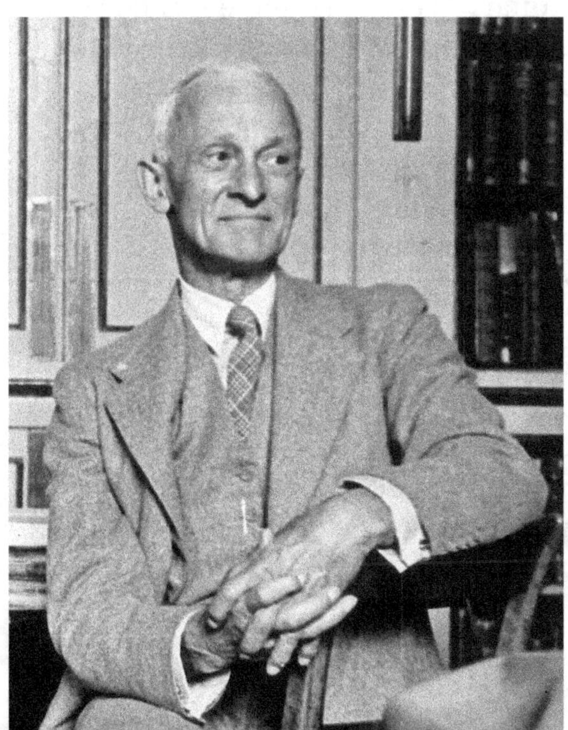

Harvey Williams Cushing

PPID

In most cases of PPID, there is no hypercortisolaemia (characteristic of Cushing's syndrome). The problem is not in the anterior lobe of the pituitary gland (characteristic of Cushing's disease), but in the intermediate lobe. Because of these two important distinctions, the scientific community agreed a long time ago that the condition should have its own name: PPID.

The acronym PPID stands for Pituitary Pars Intermedia Dysfunction:
- *Pituitary* is short for pituitary gland,
- *Pars intermedia* is the Latin name for intermediate lobe,
- *Dysfunction* is impaired or abnormal functioning of (a part of) an organ.

Although the terms 'equine Cushing's syndrome' and 'equine Cushing's disease' are also common, it is still important to use the more specific and accurate name PPID.

NEURODEGENERATION OR ENDOCRINOPATHY?

PPID is frequently referred to as an endocrinopathy. An endocrinopathy is a condition resulting from improper endocrine gland function. This malfunction, in the case of PPID, is primarily caused by the gradual deterioration of nerves connecting the hypothalamus to the pituitary gland. Thus, PPID is first and foremost a neurodegenerative condition (neuron = nerve cell, degeneration = deterioration, breakdown). For comparison, in Cushing's disease, there is no actual nerve breakdown.

Despite this clarification, you will still encounter no less than 20 hormones in this book, as ultimately, it is the overall hormonal imbalance that the horse suffers from that causes the condition identified as PPID.

DEFINITION

PPID is a neurodegenerative disorder of the hypothalamic dopamine-producing nerves that results in a loss of dopaminergic inhibition of the pituitary gland's intermediate lobe, chronic overproduction of POMC and its derived hormones, increased biological activity of these hormones, and the development of clinical signs of the condition. Pituitary gland enlargement can lead to neurological difficulties later in the disease's course.

DOPAMINERGIC
Responding to, releasing, or otherwise involving dopamine.

Simply put, the problem in PPID is that for too long, too many melanocortins circulate in the bloodstream and that the pituitary gland can swell, thus causing the clinical problems that can affect the horse.

PHYSIOLOGY, PATHOLOGY AND PATHOPHYSIOLOGY

Physiology is the science that studies the mechanisms of the functioning of living things. Pathology and pathophysiology look at where these mechanisms go wrong, where pathophysiology looks specifically at cells, tissues, organs, and the like.

DOPAMINE, POMC AND MELANOCORTINS

In horses with PPID, the quantity of dopamine-producing nerves in the hypothalamus decreases over time. As a result, less dopamine is produced, resulting in insufficient inhibition of the pituitary gland's intermediate lobe. Because of this lack of inhibition, too much of the 'raw material' POMC is formed, and as a consequence, too much of the POMC-derived hormones: ACTH, alpha-MSH, CLIP, and beta-endorphin.

Dopamine inhibits both the conversion of POMC to ACTH and the conversion of ACTH to alpha-MSH and CLIP. When there is less dopamine to inhibit these processes, more ACTH is produced from POMC. Most of this is promptly converted into alpha-MSH and CLIP. As a result, these two hormones increase first. Normally, the first conversion process (POMC to ACTH) is more strongly inhibited than the second (ACTH to alpha-MSH, CLIP). Due to the lack of inhibition, ACTH levels rise beyond the capacity for conversion into alpha-MSH and CLIP, resulting in an excess of ACTH [117].

PPID-affected horses have up to six times fewer dopamine-producing nerve endings in the intermediate lobe [177]. The amount of dopamine in the intermediate lobe of horses with PPID is eight times lower than in healthy horses of the same age [105]. Another indication of reduced dopamine production is that up to nine times fewer dopamine breakdown products (dopamine metabolites) are found in the pituitary glands of horses affected by PPID at autopsy compared to healthy age-matched horses [105].

CORTISOL

Cortisol, a hormone produced in the adrenal cortex, does inhibit ACTH secretion. This is called negative feedback. However, this inhibition happens in the pituitary gland's frontal lobe, not in the intermediate lobe. As you now know now, the latter is controlled by the hypothalamus.

While cortisol receptors are present in the intermediate lobe of the pituitary gland in rats, they are only found in the frontal lobe in horses [134].

As the intermediate lobe functions independently of the negative feedback mechanisms in the hypothalamic-pituitary-adrenal axis, it is not considered a part of this axis, even though ACTH from the intermediate lobe does have an effect on the production of cortisol by the adrenal glands [198].

> ### HYPOTHALAMIC-PITUITARY-ADRENAL AXIS
> The system of direct (neuro)-hormonal influences and feedback loops between the hypothalamus, pituitary and adrenal glands.

In humans and dogs with Cushing's disease, excessive ACTH often leads to overactive and enlarged adrenal glands. We only observe this in one out of five horses with PPID [117, 130, 203]. This usually keeps blood cortisol levels within acceptable limits as well [59, 229]. One possible reason for these two findings could be that the ACTH released by the intermediate lobe has a lower hormonal potency, also known as biological activity, in comparison to the ACTH from the frontal lobe [16, 17, 25].

CORTISOL DYSREGULATION

However, we should not get too obsessed with cortisol levels. Other abnormalities in cortisol metabolism may also be involved. This is referred to as cortisol dysregulation. Let us have a closer look at that.

FREE CORTISOL

Free cortisol, also referred to as unbound cortisol, is the biological active form that is not bound to proteins like cortisol-binding globulin (CBG) or albumin. Unbound cortisol can travel freely in the body's tissues and activate receptors. In healthy horses, around 10% of cortisol in the blood is in its unbound form [62].

A 2016 study compared horses with PPID or EMS/insulin dysregulation to healthy horses. Total cortisol levels were comparable in all horses [62]. However, overweight yet otherwise healthy horses displayed higher levels of free cortisol. Ponies with EMS exhibited higher free cortisol levels compared to horses with the same condition. The researchers believe that assessing free cortisol levels rather than total cortisol levels would be more accurate. High levels of free cortisol may explain certain clinical signs.

GLUCOCORTICOIDS

Another study found that administering ACTH to healthy horses increased not only cortisol but also other glucocorticoids such as cortisone and corticosterone [206]. This again could be an indication that we are focusing too much on cortisol alone.

TISSUE-SPECIFIC CORTISOL METABOLISM
A 2018 study questions the theory of reduced biological activity of ACTH from the intermediate lobe. The researchers proposed a different theory. They observed that enzymes involved in tissue-specific cortisol metabolism were dysregulated. This dysregulation does alter tissue exposure to glucocorticoids, but it is not reflected in cortisol measurements in the blood [59].

From studies on rats and humans, we know that a particular enzyme (11-b-HSD1) in adipose tissue can convert biologically inactive cortisone into biologically active cortisol [166, 182]. This could also explain certain clinical signs typically caused by elevated cortisol levels in the blood.

The relative amount of glucocorticoids in adipose tissue is almost four times higher in horses than in humans. The ratio between the amount of cortisol in adipose tissue and blood is also greater. Consequently, an increase in body fat might have a more significant effect on cortisol metabolism compared to that observed in humans [59].

CORTISOL METABOLITES
The 2018 study further revealed that PPID-affected horses had four times as many cortisol breakdown products (cortisol metabolites) in their urine [59]. This points to higher cortisol metabolism and clearance, which might indicate increased cortisol production.

It is logical to assume that with higher breakdown the total amount of cortisol can only remain the same if production goes up along with it. However, the researchers suggest that the opposite may be the case. The heightened cortisol production could be the body's response to counterbalance the increased cortisol clearance.

Another study found a threefold increase in cortisol metabolite excretion in obese horses without a change in their blood cortisol levels [20].

PITUITARY ENLARGEMENT
Cell enlargement (hypertrophy) and cell proliferation (hyperplasia) cause the intermediate lobe of the pituitary gland to expand, known as pituitary enlargement. At a later stage, one or more benign glandular tissue tumours (adenomas) may form.

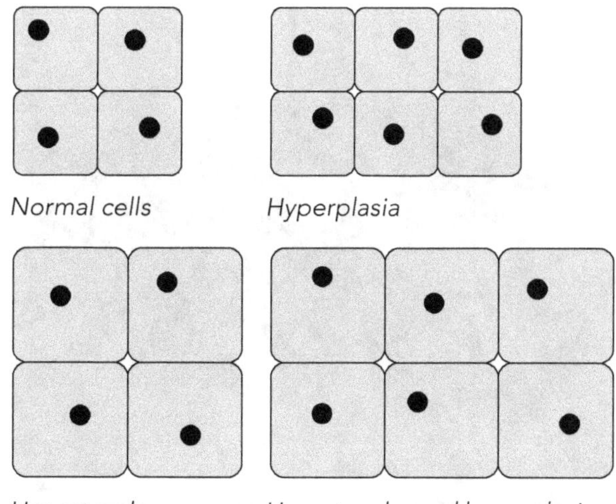

Schematic representation of pituitary enlargement

This is a consequence of the lack of inhibition. This is because the cells of the intermediate lobe do what they are supposed to do until they are inhibited without inhibition, they will continue to enlarge and multiply and subsequently increase their hormone production.

Post-mortem examinations found macroadenomas (see sidebar 'Histological classification') larger than 10 mm / 0.4 inches in diameter in nearly 70% of horses [254]. Additionally, a separate study revealed that horses in advanced stages of PPID had pituitary glands that were up to three times heavier than those of healthy horses [145].

Adenomas in the intermediate lobe have their own name: Pars Intermedia Pituitary Adenoma (PIPA).

Some of the manifestations of the disease are caused by the pressure exerted by the enlarged pituitary gland on adjacent brain structures. We will go into these neurological issues later in the chapter.

The hypothalamus can also come under compression from the pituitary gland. Within the pituitary itself, the same is true for the anterior and posterior lobes, which come under pressure as the intermediate lobe claims more space.

While some people may think of an adenoma as a cancerous tumour, this is not accurate. Adenoma cells do not multiply quickly, and they do not spread to other parts of the body, a process known as metastasis.

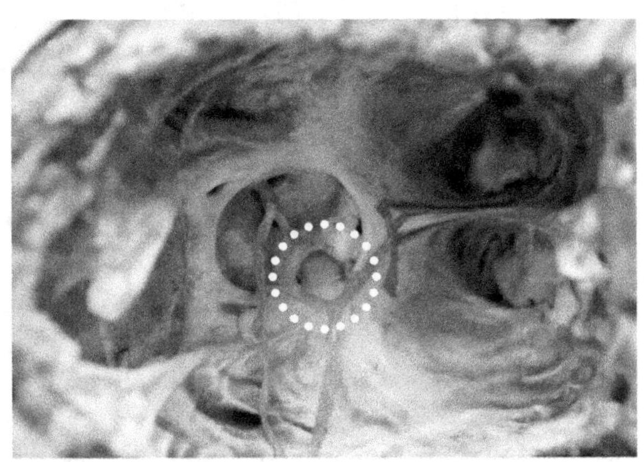

Healthy pituitary gland

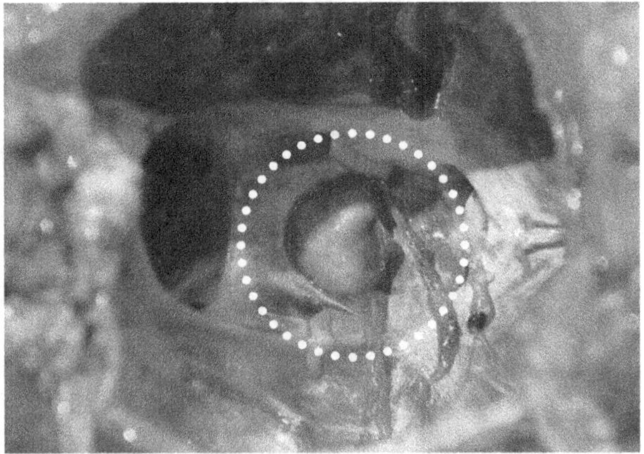

Pituitary gland, grade 5
(photos: Zefanja Vermeulen)

HISTOLOGICAL CLASSIFICATION

In science, the state of the pituitary intermediate lobe in PPID-affected horses is classified using a grading system:

- Grade 1. Normal
- Grade 2. Moderate hypertrophy/hyperplasia in one or more locations in the intermediate lobe
- Grade 3. Hyperplasia of the whole intermediate lobe
- Grade 4. As grade 3, with at least one micro-adenoma (1-5 mm / 0.04-0.2 inches in diameter)
- Grade 5. As grade 4, with at least one macro-adenoma (more than 5 mm / 0.2 inches in diameter)

Grade 2 is still considered part of the normal ageing process. Horses at this stage typically show no clinical signs and have normal hormone levels.

Grades 3, 4 and 5 correspond to mild, moderate, and severe PPID, respectively. The number and severity of clinical signs increase with each grade, as do the changes in the blood count. No horse can avoid the PPID diagnosis by grade 5.

A 1997 study found adenomas and enlarged pituitary glands (grade 4) in a number of horses during autopsy, without those horses having shown any clinical signs of PPID [146]. The enlarged pituitary gland could be explained by the fact that its size is subject to seasonal variation. A 2011 study showed that the intermediate lobe – and therefore the whole pituitary gland – is larger in autumn compared to non-autumnal months [74].

CLINICAL SIGNS

PPID itself is not a painful condition. It is the clinical signs that cause pain and discomfort. The better you monitor the development of clinical signs and treat them, the higher your horse's quality of life will be.

A clinical sign that was not there before and suddenly presents itself could mean that the PPID is progressing. Consider retesting and adjusting medication. In the upcoming chapters, we will cover blood tests and medication in detail.

Take photos of your horse on a regular basis and keep a journal to record changes in its health, condition, appearance, and behaviour.

It is becoming increasingly clear that horses with PPID can have a wide range of clinical problems. We also now know that PPID often shows few or very subtle signs of disease in the early stages.

It has taken a while to develop this knowledge base because the results of scientific studies are often based on small numbers of horses, where the disease was already advanced. In addition, for ethical reasons we obviously cannot induce PPID in otherwise healthy horses for experimental study purposes.

The fact that PPID often afflicts older horses, with a range of other ailments and age-related problems, has also clouded our ability to study PPID independently of these other conditions.

Let us take a look at what we know about how PPID manifests itself.

The three most common clinical signs of PPID are hypertrichosis (a form of excess hair growth), laminitis and muscle atrophy (reduced muscle mass) of the shoulders, withers, back and glutes, followed by behavioural change and weight loss [102].

These clinical signs are of course not PPID-specific, although hypertrichosis is the closest exception to this rule, obviously, your veterinarian will take this into account. They will consider the entire clinical picture, which again, can vary greatly between individual animals. In part, this can be explained by differences in the melanocortin composition and biological activity,

the time of year, the extent to which the adrenal glands are involved in the disease, the presence or absence of EMS/insulin dysregulation (which will be discussed in detail later), and the horse's age [197].

SEASONAL RISE

Most, if not all, hormone-related clinical signs follow to a greater or lesser extent the rise in autumn of ACTH, its derived hormones alpha-MSH and CLIP, and possibly beta-endorphin.

Even if your horse is receiving the drug pergolide, it is still susceptible to the hormonal effect of this seasonal rise. It is therefore worth noting that some clinical signs may suddenly return in the autumn to a mild degree.

COAT CHANGES

Because you see your horse every day, you can spot this property of PPID better and earlier than the veterinarian. Owner-reported coat changes are more predictive than hypertrichosis diagnosed by the vet [214]. Therefore, mention this when they come by for diagnosis; especially if your horse has been clipped not so long ago. After all, the vet cannot know what the unshaved version of your horse looked like.

The exact cause of coat changes is still uncertain. It was long assumed to be the pressure exerted by the enlarged pituitary gland on the heat-regulating part of the hypothalamus. Hormones like alpha-MSH, cortisol, melatonin, testosterone, and prolactin have been considered culprits, but there is no strong scientific evidence to support these ideas. Notably, since coat changes affect mares and geldings as frequently as stallions, we can rule out testosterone as a cause.

DELAYED SHEDDING, COAT DISCOLOURATION

Delayed or irregular shedding and coat discolouration are often the first signs of coat changes you see in your horse. In rustic breeds, which usually have a thick winter coat, you are more likely to notice that shedding is more difficult. Coat discolouration is more likely to be seen in horses with darker coats. Where coat discolouration is a precursor, problems with shedding are already features of hypertrichosis. This is one of the clinical signs that horse owners can frequently misinterpret as a normal part of aging.

HYPERTRICHOSIS

In hypertrichosis, we see abnormally thick, curly and long hair. While the precise cause remains a mystery, we do know it disrupts the hair growth cycle, causing hair follicles to stay in the growth phase for an extended period, sometimes permanently [31].

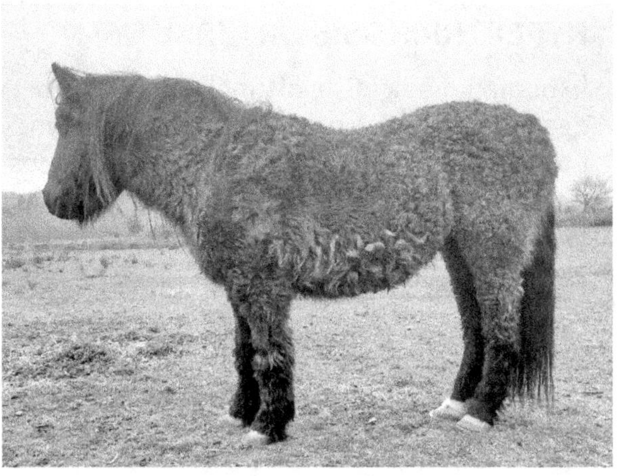

Advanced hypertrichosis

Hypertrichosis is the most distinctive sign of PPID, found in nearly 70% of affected horses [102].

Hypertrichosis usually starts under the jaw, the underside of the neck, the legs, and behind the elbows. The coat may appear duller and feel coarser or thicker than usual. Subsequently, it spreads to the rest of the body. In breeds with a thin coat, the latter may not always occur, meaning it can take longer to notice the presence of hypertrichosis.

In donkeys, especially long-haired breeds, changes in the coat are less noticeable. This is because donkeys have longer and thicker coats compared to horses. Additionally, donkeys shed their winter coat more slowly in the spring than horses, so it is common to see remnants of the winter coat even in the summer.

> ## HYPERTRICHOSIS OR HIRSUTISM?
>
> In human medicine, a distinction is made between hypertrichosis and hirsutism. Both terms describe excessive hair growth. However, they are not the same. In hypertrichosis, hair grows more than one would expect, in places where hair normally grows. In hirsutism, the hair grows in places where it normally would not or hardly at all. For example, the excessive facial hair growth that can occur in women.
>
> Hypertrichosis in humans typically stems from hereditary factors or medication use. Hirsutism, on the other hand, is mainly triggered by hormonal imbalances. In particular, an excess of male hormones (androgens) or heightened sensitivity of hair follicles to these hormones. This clinical sign can be seen by women who have Cushing's disease.
>
> For many years, veterinary medicine did not differentiate between Cushing's disease and PPID, so the term hirsutism was also used in the context of PPID. However, when referring to excessive hair growth in horses with PPID, we now use the term hypertrichosis.

HYPER- OR HYPOHIDROSIS

Hyperhidrosis refers to excessive sweating. In equines affected by PPID, this excessive sweating is mostly observed on the neck and shoulders. As with coat changes, scientists have not fully understood why this happens. It may, in part, be a response to the long coat. Yet there are horses that continue to sweat after being shaved or that sweat at low ambient temperatures.

It could also be due to the enlarged pituitary gland pressing on the hypothalamus. Science is also looking into high beta-endorphin levels in the blood as a potential cause.

Hypohidrosis is when a horse does not sweat enough, making it hard for them to cool down. This can lead to elevated body temperature, increased heart rate and respiratory rate. This condition can be particularly problematic in the summer when the horse needs to regulate body heat efficiently.

POLYURIA AND POLYDIPSIA

A significant proportion of equines with PPID suffer from insulin dysregulation (abnormalities in insulin metabolism). One of the consequences of this is increased glucose levels in the blood (hyperglycaemia). Some of the glucose enters the urine. This is called glycosuria. Glucose retains fluid, causing the horse to urinate more (polyuria) and, as a result, to drink more (polydipsia).

Elevated cortisol levels in PPID-affected horses may be a secondary factor contributing to polyuria. Cortisol inhibits the hormone ADH (antidiuretic hormone), which plays a role in stimulating water absorption by the kidneys, reducing the amount of water that ends up in the urine. Inhibition of ADH leads to increased water excretion in the urine. Additionally, less ADH is being produced due to the pressure from the enlarged intermediate lobe of the pituitary gland on the part of the posterior lobe where ADH is stored and released into the bloodstream. These factors collectively contribute to polyuria in horses with PPID [207].

The combination of polyuria and polydipsia is a significant clinical manifestation in horses with both PPID and EMS/insulin dysregulation, impacting around 30% of such cases [117]. In donkeys, polyuria and polydipsia tend to be less common than in horses and ponies.

> EMS
>> Equine metabolic syndrome. A cluster of interrelated metabolic problems.
>
> INSULIN DYSREGULATION (ID)
>> Overarching term for abnormalities in insulin metabolism. In particular, hyperinsulinaemia and insulin resistance.

Polyuria is more noticeable in stabled horses due to quicker soiling of the stable. With horses in pasture, where you as the owner have to refill the water yourself, polydipsia is more noticeable

because you have to do this much more frequently. Water consumption can easily double.

ADIPOSITY

Adiposity is a type of overweight characterised by an abnormal fat distribution across the body. Fat bumps above the eyes are particularly common in PPID-afflicted horses, an area which in older, healthy horses, on the contrary, tends to follow out. Fat may also accumulate under the lower eyelid, resulting in a swollen appearance of the eyes. Owners say that the horse seems to look out of its eyes differently than before. Other areas where fat may accumulate include the top of the shoulders, the trunk, the tail head, the sheath (in males), or udder (in mares). Adiposity is a component of EMS. The cresty neck, often seen in EMS cases, is not a typical feature in PPID-affected horses who do not have this metabolic disorder.

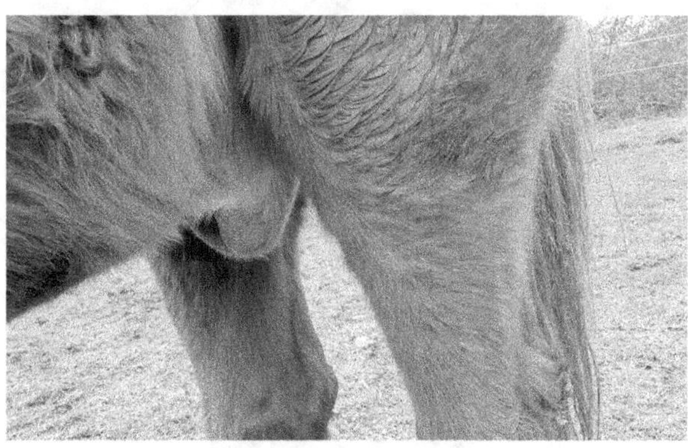

Swollen sheath due to adiposity

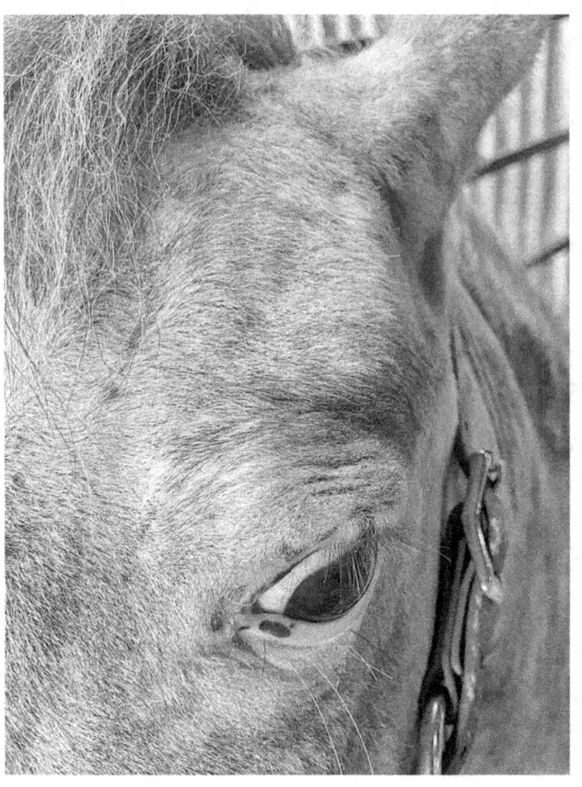

Fat deposits above the eyes
(photo: Donna Nyland)

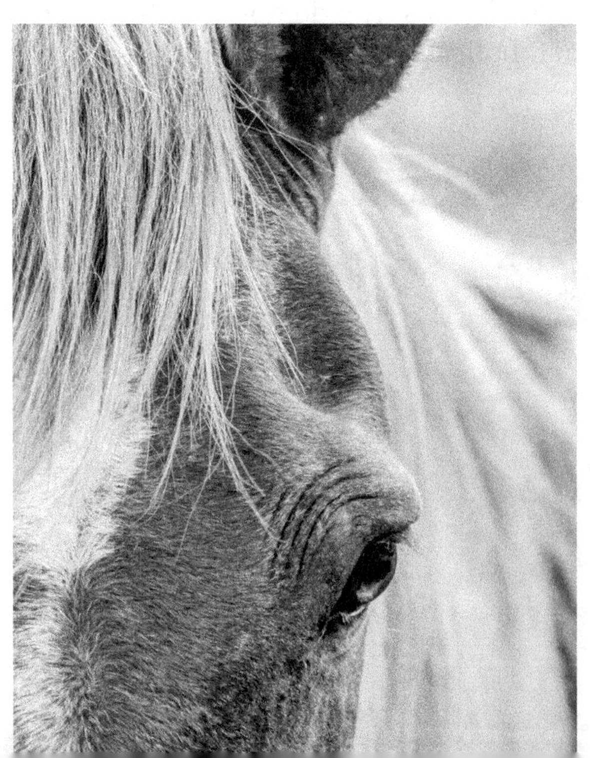

Hollows above the eye sockets
in a senior without adiposity
(photo: Rodolfo Quirós)

As mentioned earlier, alpha-MSH is responsible for accumulating fat reserves, preparing horses for winter. This survival mechanism is associated with adiposity and obesity in horses with PPID, whether they have EMS/insulin dysregulation or not.

WEIGHT LOSS

Dental problems can lead to pain during chewing as well as to quidding, where the horse drops partially chewed food. This discomfort can result in reduced food intake, contributing to weight loss. Besides weight loss due a decrease in body fat, PPID-affected horses also lose weight due to muscle loss (atrophy). Dental problems and muscle loss are discussed later in this chapter.

INCREASED APPETITE

Despite weight loss, horses with PPID typically maintain a normal appetite. In some cases, there may even be an increased appetite. When this heightened appetite becomes extreme, it is referred to as hyperphagia. This increased appetite could result from leptin resistance, detailed in the sidebar on page 44.

BEHAVIOURAL CHANGE

Horses with PPID often show a calmer demeanour, at times bordering on apathy. Their willingness to work may decline, a condition referred to as exercise intolerance. This ranks as the fourth most common clinical sign, affecting just over 40% of PPID-affected horses.

Apathy and decreased willingness to work are characteristics commonly observed in various chronic conditions, not just PPID. Horses with PPID are often described as docile and more tolerant of pain, which is attributed to their notably higher beta-endorphin levels, sometimes up to 60 times higher. Beta-endorphins primarily function as pain suppressants, and in horses afflicted by PPID, the biological activity of beta-endorphins is thought to be higher than in healthy horses [105, 197].

It cannot be ruled out that lower dopamine production also has a direct effect on behaviour. Dopamine is involved in the body's reward system, so a decrease in dopamine could result in fewer hormonal rewards and could therefore potentially lead to behavioural changes. However, at present, this connection between dopamine levels and behaviour in horses with PPID remains largely theoretical and requires further research to establish a concrete link.

Some clinical signs or complications can also be seen as stand-alone conditions that cause behavioural changes. For example, apathy is associated with insulin resistance [117].

Exercise intolerance should not be confused with subclinical laminitis. Subclinical laminitis may involve mild pain, which can significantly reduce a horse's inclination to exercise.

MUSCLE ATROPHY

In nearly half of horses with PPID muscle atrophy (or muscle loss) is a common occurrence [102]. This condition involves the thinning and weakening of the muscles. Initially, the shoulders and back show signs of declining musculature, followed by the withers and buttocks. In more advanced stages, the abdominal muscles also weaken, leading to the development of the characteristic pot belly appearance.

Muscle atrophy is believed to result from an imbalance in protein production and a breakdown in muscle tissue. While the exact mechanisms are not yet fully understood, glucocorticoids are considered prime suspects in this process. Glucocorticoids are known to accelerate the breakdown of proteins, leading to muscle atrophy [224]. PPID-affected horses show an elevation in the enzyme MuRF-1, known for its involvement in protein breakdown in muscle tissue [169]. Glucocorticoids stimulate this enzyme. Insulin resistance and chronic inflammation may also play a role in muscle breakdown [233].

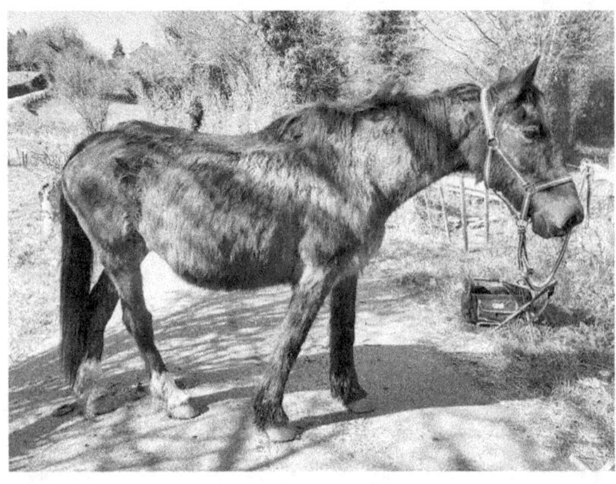

Pot belly due to muscle atrophy

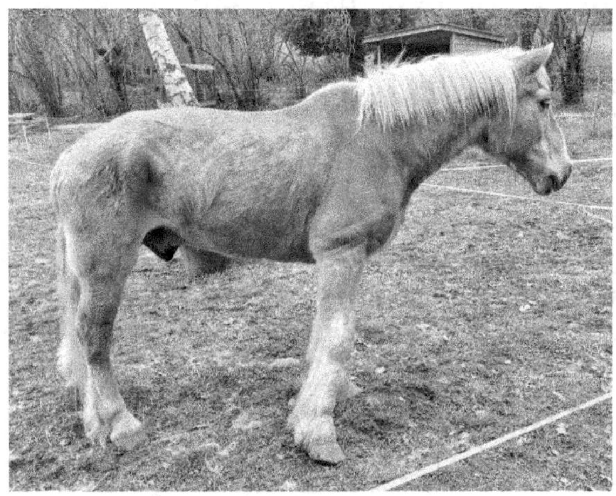

Advanced muscle atrophy,
without pot belly

While muscle loss is also a common feature of aging in horses, it should still be considered an important clinical manifestation of PPID. The key difference is that in natural aging, muscle loss generally happens gradually. In contrast, in horses with PPID, muscle atrophy occurs at a much faster rate.

Depending on the breed, physical condition, and degree of overweight, initial signs of muscle loss may be overlooked at first. A lumpy appearance of the fat layer in overweight horses is an indication that the underlying muscles are atrophying.

If you still ride your horse, it is essential to pay close attention to any signs of reduced musculature. It would be unfair to ask your horse to carry you when it is no longer physically capable of doing so due to muscle loss.

TENDON AND LIGAMENT LAXITY
Tendons and ligaments can weaken. Problems with the suspensory ligament, particularly in the hind legs, are a common issue in horses with PPID. This unfortunately often lead to euthanasia, due to the poor response of this painful condition to analgesic drugs.

In horses with suspensory ligament issues, a noticeable sign can be the hyperextension of the fetlock, where this joint descends too far. This is somewhat similar to the connective tissue degeneration seen in people with Cushing's disease or after prolonged high-dose synthetic corticosteroid treatment [241]. Achilles tendon rupture is more common in these people [239].

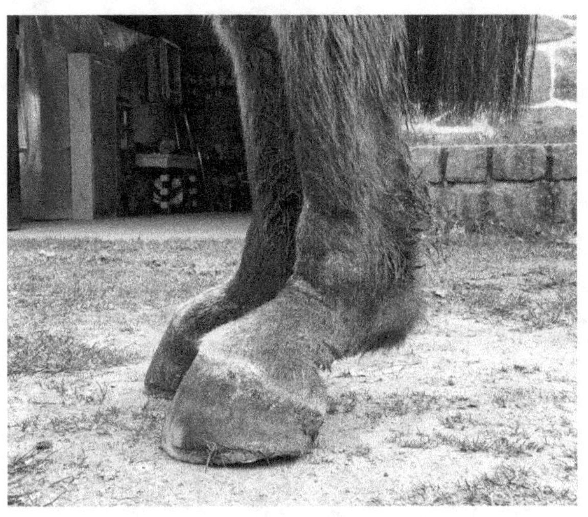

Hyperextension

We believe degeneration of the suspensory ligament is caused by cortisol. Although cortisol levels are not structurally elevated in horses with PPID, too much free cortisol in the blood may still contribute to the degeneration of tendons and ligaments (see page 24) [62]. Additionally, there is evidence to suggest that tissue-specific cortisol metabolism in tendons and ligaments plays a role in this process (see page 25) [12].

There seems to be a link between insulin dysregulation and ESPA (Equine Systemic Proteoglycan Accumulation) in Peruvian pasos and their cross-breeds [241]. ESPA is a connective tissue disorder that is more prevalent in this breed. Whether this link can be extended to other breeds with insulin dysregulation remains an open question.

However, what is certain is that under the microscope, remarkable similarities can be observed in tissue samples from the tendons and ligaments of PPID-affected horses with abnormal sagging fetlocks, horses with ESPA, and people with Achilles tendon ruptures.

OPPORTUNISTIC INFECTIONS AND IMMUNE PROBLEMS

INFECTIONS AND INFLAMMATION

Horses with PPID are usually older, and as horses age, their immune defences decline. This characteristic of ageing is called immunosenescence [147]. Inflammatory activity in the body also increases with age. We call this 'inflamm-aging'. It is a characteristic of the aging process in which various factors, including the elevated presence of pro-inflammatory cytokines (proteins), contribute to a state of low-grade inflammation in the body [144].

> **LOW-GRADE INFLAMMATION**
> Chronic state of inflammation of the body, without visible signs of inflammation.

Interestingly, this low-grade inflammation or silent inflammation is often more prevalent in healthy horses than in horses with PPID [47]. This difference could potentially be explained by the anti-inflammatory effects of the hormones alpha-MSH and beta-endorphin, which are involved in regulating inflammation and may thus have a protective role in the context of PPID [93].

Certain pro-inflammatory cytokines make horses more susceptible to bacterial infections. Interleukin-8 (IL-8) is an example of such a cytokine. In horses with PPID, blood IL-8 concentrations are elevated [47, 78].

Chronic inflammation is also partially linked to insulin resistance. Given that at least one in three PPID-affected horses also experiences insulin dysregulation and, consequently, insulin resistance, this is an important factor to consider.

INSULIN RESISTANCE
Physiological condition in which cells fail to respond to the normal actions of insulin.

Alpha-MSH, beta-endorphin and cortisol also suppress immune responses. As a result, infections and inflammations might be present but go unnoticed. For example, traces of chronic lung infection (pneumonia) or bladder infection (cystitis) are regularly found at autopsy, even though the horse had not exhibited any noticeable signs while alive [130].

The infections and inflammations most often found by the vet in PPID-afflicted horses are rain rot (dermatophilosis), mud fever (pastern dermatitis), sinus infection (sinusitis), pink eye (conjunctivitis), eye infection (uveitis), gum inflammation (gingivitis), lung infection (pneumonia), bladder infection (cystitis), uterine infection (uteritis), and hoof abscesses.

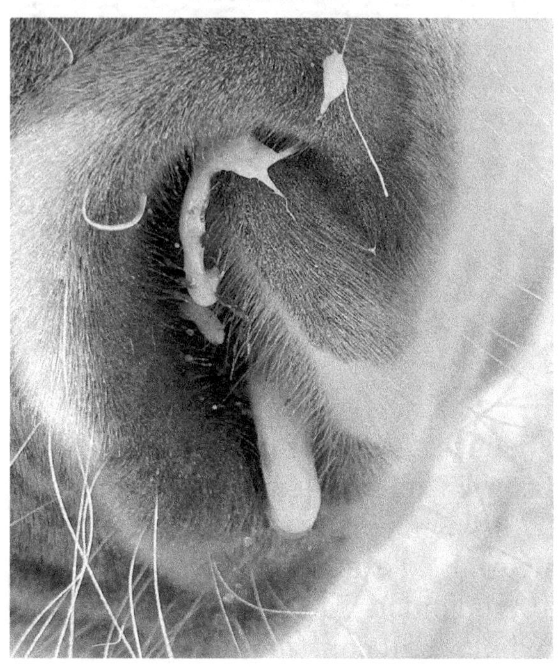

Sinusitis

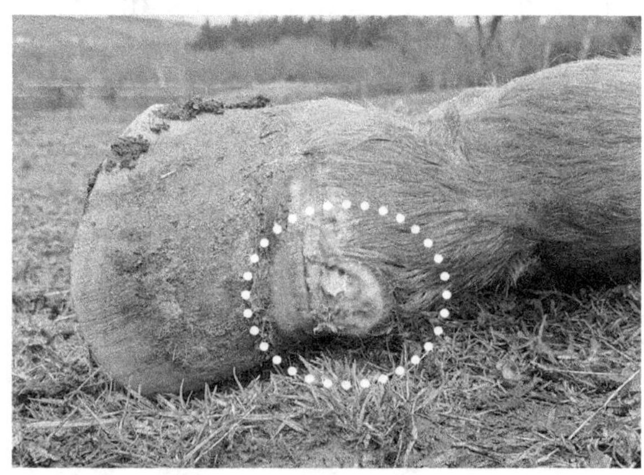

Coronary band abscess

Whilst in the early stages of PPID, the horse can suffer from ligament inflammation (desmitis), tendon inflammation (tendinitis) or inflammation of the tendon sheath (tendovaginitis). As mentioned earlier, horses with PPID are more prone to tendon and ligament weakness and in some cases, these horses can develop both problems.

The toxins released by inflammation activate platelets that form clots (microthromboses) in the capillaries of the hoof, clogging them. In addition, the platelets release the hormone serotonin that constricts blood vessels. Vessel blockage and vasoconstriction restrict blood flow to important tissues in the hooves. This reduced blood flow can contribute to the onset of laminitis or worsen an existing case of laminitis.

Laminitis caused by toxins is called SIRS-related laminitis (or sepsis-related). This is not the same as endocrinopathic laminitis which you will read about later and which is typical of PPID. So, inflammation can contribute to laminitis through a different pathway.

IMPAIRED WOUND HEALING

Wound healing is generally slower in older horses and especially in those with PPID.

Additionally, some horses with PPID may experience lower sensitivity in the cornea of the eye [127]. These factors, in combination with the natural effects of aging and increased levels of melanocortins in the blood, can contribute to impaired wound healing. This impaired wound healing can increase the risk of non-healing or recurrent corneal ulcers.

MORE SUSCEPTIBLE TO WORM INFESTATION, HIGHER EGG COUNT IN FAECES

Horses with PPID often exhibit a higher egg count (the number of worm eggs) in their manure, which indicates that they are more susceptible to worm infestations. Furthermore, these infestations are typically more severe in horses with PPID compared to those without the condition.

It is not yet known what mechanism is responsible for the increased susceptibility to parasites. While lowered resistance and increased susceptibility to infections may be plausible factors contributing to this vulnerability, it is worth noting that a 2010 study did not observe a direct correlation between the risk of parasite infestation and increasing age alone in horses [132].

INAPPROPRIATE MILK PRODUCTION

Mares may encounter issues with milk yield, showing either continued secretion after the foal is weaned or milk engorgement in mares not currently raising a foal, often referred to as witch's milk. Another possible cause is an udder infection (mastitis). As you now know, horses with PPID are more prone to this kind of problem.

The issue might stem from an excess of the hormone prolactin produced in the anterior lobe (i.c. the tubular lobe, (see page 16) of the pituitary gland. Exactly how PPID affects prolactin concentration, is unclear, however, the secretion of prolactin, like that of melanocortins, is inhibited by dopamine [58] and therefore the dopamine deficit in mares with PPID could cause too much prolactin to be produced [190].

IRREGULAR OESTRUS, INFERTILITY

As mares age, they are more likely to experience irregular oestrous cycles and may face increased difficulty in conceiving or may even fail to conceive. This failure to conceive may be even higher in mares with PPID, than in healthy, older mares.

The cause is thought to be reduced dopaminergic inhibition of key reproductive hormones. As mentioned earlier, prolactin inhibits ovulation. Hence, if dopamine fails to adequately regulate prolactin, ovulation inhibition becomes more pronounced.

Another contributing factor might be the reduced production of the reproductive hormones FSH (follicle stimulating hormone) and LH (luteinising hormone). This reduction is due to the inhibitory effect that certain adrenal cortical hormones (androgens) have on them. At a later stage, hormone production decreases as a result of the pressure exerted by the enlarged intermediate lobe of the pituitary on the anterior lobe, where these hormones are produced [104].

While most studies indicate that blood cortisol levels typically do not significantly increase in PPID, a specific study on the relationship between PPID and infertility in broodmares did find elevated cortisol levels (hypercortisolaemia) [225]. Cortisol has an inhibitory effect on the anterior lobe of the pituitary gland.

In addition, EMS/insulin dysregulation is associated with reproductive problems [66]. Obesity, elevated insulin and leptin levels, along with pro-inflammatory cytokines, can all contribute to reduced fertility in mares. Since a proportion of PPID-affected horses also have EMS/insulin dysregulation, this is a factor to consider.

Additionally, horses with PPID are more susceptible to inflammation, including chronic uterine infection, which can be a contributing factor in infertility.

SWOLLEN SHEATH AND ACCUMULATION OF SMEGMA

Males also encounter specific PPID-related issues. As stated earlier, body fat can accumulate in the penile sheath. This causes a swollen appearance of the sheath. However, a more critical concern arises from this swelling, as it impedes the proper drainage of smegma, leading to the formation of hard lumps known as beans. These beans can obstruct the urinary tract, with evidenciary unpleasant consequences.

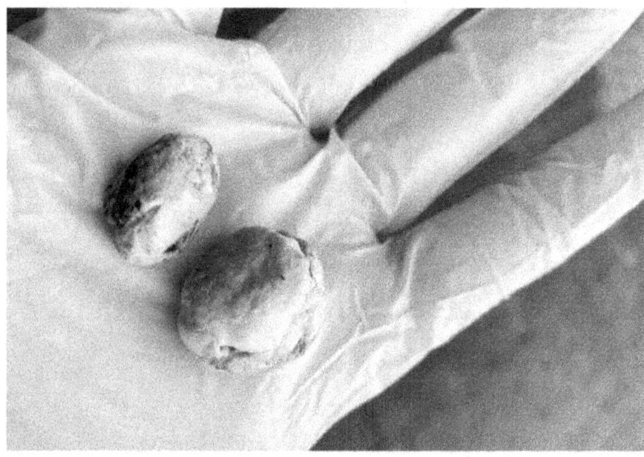

Beans
(photo: Kady Mauro)

The smegma that does come out of the sheath is typically dark, malodorous and may leave greasy marks on the inner hind legs. In geldings, accumulation of smegma is more common than in stallions, as the penis is less likely to come out of the sheath completely. Without regular cleaning of the sheath, there is an increased risk of infection

NEUROLOGICAL PROBLEMS

Neurological issues typically appear in the advanced stages of the disease the result of enlargement of the intermediate lobe of the pituitary gland; a clinical sign that typically occurs only later in the disease progression as it causes the pituitary gland as a whole to become larger. The enlarged pituitary gland exerts pressure on surrounding brain tissue, leading to conditions such as blindness, seizures, narcolepsy (irrepressible sleep attacks), and ataxia (muscle dysfunction). In the case of blindness, for example, the pituitary presses on the part of the brain where the optic nerves cross: the chiasma opticum. Fortunately, these problems are not common, as they impose a significant burden on the horse.

OSTEOPOROSIS

Osteoporosis is advanced demineralisation (decalcification) of bone tissue, resulting in a deterioration of bone quality and an increased risk of fractures. Osteoporosis is already more common in older horses, but can additionally occur as a complication of PPID, with the imbalance in cortisol levels as the suspected cause.

Statistics reveal an above-average euthanasia rate for horses with PPID due to pelvic, rib, jaw and coffin bone fractures [203].

Another concern is that the surface area of the coffin bone becomes smaller due to osteoporosis. This reduces the bonding area between this bone and the hoof wall, potentially exacerbating laminitis.

DENTAL PROBLEMS/EOTRH

The acronym EOTRH stands for Equine Odontoclastic Tooth Resorption and Hypercementosis.

- *Equine* pertains to horses
- *Odontoclasts* are cells responsible for the resorption (dissolution) of dental tissues
- *Hypercementosis* is the excessive deposition of cementum, a bone-like substance that covers and protects the tooth root's entire surface while anchoring it into the jawbone beneath the gumline.

EOTRH is a dental condition that primarily affects older horses. It leads to a breakdown or loosening or inflammation in the surrounding tissues of the incisors and canines in particular. Over time, the roots of multiple teeth gradually dissolve. In an attempt to stabilise these teeth or combat infections, the body deposits additional cementum around the roots (hypercementosis). Bacterial infections can easily take hold in these affected teeth, potentially causing abscesses. The teeth may become loose or even break. In severe cases, EOTRH can extend to the jawbone, resulting in bone inflammation (osteitis) [248].

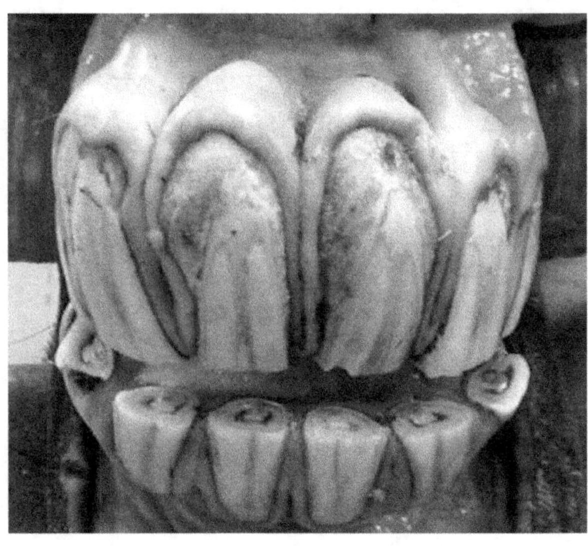

EOTRH
(photo: Cedric Coucke)

EOTRH is a slowly progressing disease of which we do not yet fully understand the causes. Overloading between upper and lower teeth due to misalignment and prolonged hard feeding could play a role.

There is some indication that horses with PPID or EMS are at greater risk of developing EOTRH, however, it is also possible that EOTRH and PPID are two stand-alone conditions affection an older horse.

Because it is a painful condition, difficulties in eating will often occur, with a resulting lack of appetite and weight loss; often accompanied by excessive saliva production. Bacterial toxins can enter the bloodstream, which can cause infections in other organs.

In the next section we will investigate the theory that toxins could also indirectly be a partial cause of PPID.

Depending on the severity of the condition, it may be necessary to have the affected teeth pulled. Most horses can effectively chew grass and hay using their molars, provided these teeth remain in good condition. With only their lips and tongue, they can still graze and eat hay remarkably skilfully. It is important that the dentist regularly checks the remaining teeth and ensures good oral hygiene by removing tartar.

EMS/INSULIN DYSREGULATION

A notable proportion of horses with PPID also present with EMS/insulin dysregulation. This comorbidity is linked to a higher likelihood of developing laminitis and unfortunately a less favourable prognosis [210, 237].

INSULIN DYSREGULATION

The complex of processes in which insulin plays a role is called insulin metabolism. Insulin dysregulation (ID) encompasses any abnormalities in insulin metabolism, including hyperinsulinaemia (HI), characterised by excessive insulin in the blood, and insulin resistance (IR), where cells don't respond to insulin properly. While our focus was primarily on insulin resistance in the past, there's now a growing interest in hyperinsulinaemia and the body's insulin response to food.

Insulin dysregulation is the primary and central hormonal anomaly in EMS [156]. That is why in this book we refer to them together as EMS/insulin dysregulation (or EMS/ID), unless we are talking specifically about an element of one or the other.

After a horse consumes food high in rapidly digestible sugars and starches, there is an rise in blood sugar levels (glycaemia). In response, the body secretes insulin, a hormone produced by the pancreas. Insulin's role is to facilitate the uptake of sugar from the bloodstream into body cells. The pancreas maintains the production of insulin until blood sugar levels return to their normal range [156].

> **PANCREAS**
> Mixed gland in the duodenum that secretes hormones, including insulin, to promote the breakdown of certain nutrients.

Following food intake, the small intestine releases hormones known as incretins (GLP-1 and GIP), which in turn stimulate the pancreas to produce insulin [86]. Prolonged heightened production of these incretins may lead to hyperplasia (cellular proliferation) of the pancreatic beta cells responsible for insulin production, ultimately contributing to hyperinsulinaemia [156].

There are insulin receptors on the cell walls of muscle cells in particular, but also fat and connective tissue cells. Insulin 'instructs' the cells through these receptors, that they need to uptake and process sugar. If there is too much sugar in the blood too often, so therefore increased levels of insulin. Prolonged hyperinsulinaemia can lead to a reduced responsiveness of the receptors over time, resulting in insulin resistance [157].

HYPERGLYCAEMIA

Too much sugar now remains in the blood. This is referred to as hyperglycaemia. The horse, unable to have access to this sugar, becomes hungry and increases its food intake. Unfortunately, this serves only to exacerbate the issue as more sugar and insulin enter the bloodstream.

The excess sugar is then stored as either fat or muscle glycogen. In rare cases, an additional phase may arise where the pancreas encounters difficulty in producing sufficient insulin [48].

INSULIN CLEARANCE

Besides elevated insulin production, there may also be impaired breakdown and removal of insulin by the liver and kidneys, known as insulin clearance, that contributes to hyperinsulinaemia and, in the longer term, to insulin resistance [170].

Reduced insulin clearance by the liver can be due, among other things, to a fatty liver (hepatic steatosis), which, in turn, results from obesity and insulin dysregulation. A vicious circle, in other words. It is important to note that impaired insulin clearance is not regarded as a primary cause of hyperinsulinaemia in horses.

HYPERCORTISOLAEMIA

In PPID-affected horses with hypercortisolaemia, more proteins and fats are converted to glucose in the liver. Additionally, cortisol diminishes the insulin sensitivity of tissues, leading to reduced glucose uptake. This contributes to the development or worsening of insulin dysregulation [135]. The 2016 study mentioned earlier, found that horses with hyperinsulinaemia had elevated levels of free cortisol in their bloodstream [62].

IRON

An excess of the trace element iron in a horse's body may contribute to the development or exacerbation of hyperinsulinaemia [171], and insulin resistance [208]. Furthermore, in the case of hyperinsulinaemia, excess iron is stored in the liver [171]. Iron excess and insulin resistance, therefore, mutually reinforce each other, creating a cycle of cause and effect.

HYPERINSULINAEMIA AND LAMINITIS

Several studies demonstrate that hyperinsulinaemia, even in the absence of insulin resistance, is a significant predictor of laminitis. In these experiments, inducing hyperinsulinaemia at normal blood sugar levels resulted in laminitis in the test animals [109, 110, 151].

> *Hyperinsulinaemia (HI) and insulin resistance (IR) are typically interconnected, mutually reinforcing conditions. IR exacerbates HI, while HI contributes to the development or exacerbation of IR.*

EMS

Insulin dysregulation is a pivotal component of EMS (Equine Metabolic Syndrome). EMS is a collection of disorders. Aside from insulin dysregulation, these include body weight problems (especially adiposity), hypertension, elevated blood fat levels (hyperlipidaemia), and abnormal adipokine concentrations (see sidebar on the next page). All these aspects of EMS are known to play a role in the development of laminitis.

Horses can have a normal body weight and still have EMS. The opposite also applies [60, 70]. In other words, EMS does not always equate to being overweight, nor does being overweight necessarily imply EMS.

EMS is the result of an interaction between genetic predisposition and environmental factors. The risk of laminitis depends on how these two relate [222]. Nevertheless, the precise contribution of genetic factors to EMS development remains unclear.

What we do know is that there are horses in whom EMS, genetically speaking, hangs over their heads like a thundercloud. Even a minor change in their living conditions can shift the balance unfavourably for them.

At the other end of the spectrum, we find horses with very low genetic predisposition. Yet they are not necessarily free of risk. Encouraged in the wrong direction for long enough with feed full of rapidly digestible sugars and starches, they too can develop EMS. In fact, a group of leading scientists argue that this could be the case for any horse, including those with zero predisposition [222].

If we go by the most favourable statistics, insulin dysregulation is present in one in three horses with PPID [223]. While PPID is more prevalent in older horses, insulin dysregulation and EMS can manifest at any age and are more frequently diagnosed in younger horses.

Ponies and donkeys generally have lower insulin sensitivity compared to horses, which is why they are overrepresented in the group of PPID-afflicted equines with insulin dysregulation.

LEPTIN, LEPTIN DYSREGULATION AND ADIPONECTIN

LEPTIN

Following food intake, the hormone leptin is released from adipose tissue (body fat) and transported via the blood into the brain. There, it binds to leptin receptors on the walls of hypothalamic cells, prompting the hypothalamus to reduce food intake and increase metabolism. In contrast, if little leptin binds to the receptors, the signal will be to eat more in order maintain body weight. The metabolism then slows. Leptin thus regulates the balance between appetite and satiety.

LEPTIN DYSREGULATION

Leptin is an adipokine. Adipokines are hormones produced by fat cells. The greater the horse's body fat mass, the higher the level of leptin in the blood [83]. Prolonged high levels of leptin, referred to as hyperleptinaemia, can make the leptin receptors less responsive, leading to a state known as leptin resistance. In this condition, leptin circulates in the blood, but the hypothalamus does not respond effectively to it.

The horse eats more than it can metabolise, potentially causing or worsening obesity, adiposity, and insulin resistance. Hyperleptinaemia and leptin resistance are collectively referred to as leptin dysregulation, a component of EMS.

ADIPONECTIN

Adiponectin is an adipokine that enhances insulin sensitivity. As such, it is one of the hormones responsible for maintaining optimal blood sugar levels. It also has anti-inflammatory properties.

Horses with EMS produce less adiponectin. This so-called hypo-adiponectinaemia can result in the worsening of insulin resistance or its onset [210].

Older horses have lower adiponectin levels compared to their younger counterparts [7].

In healthy horses, leptin and adiponectin are in balance. In horses that are overweight, either obese or subject to adiposity, an overproduction of adiponectin can create a hormonal imbalance.

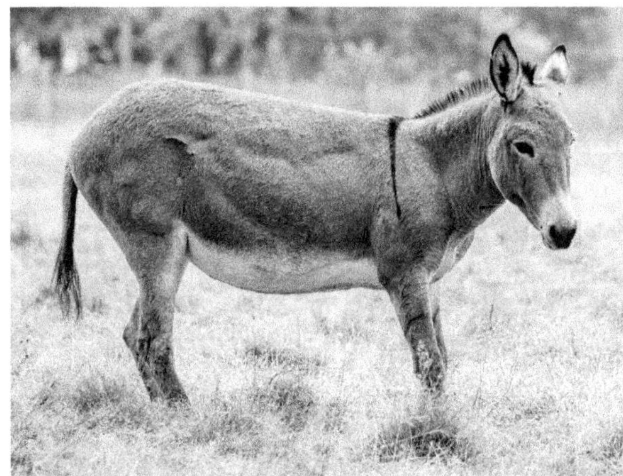

A donkey with severe overweight due to insulin dysregulation
(photo: David Selbert)

EMS VS. PPID

The question is whether EMS can make an animal more susceptible to developing PPID and vice versa, or whether the two conditions are unrelated. Presently, the scientific community has not definitively answered this question. It is possible that both conditions could exist in the same animal. It might be that PPID alone may not directly cause insulin dysregulation, and laminitis only occurs when PPID develops in an animal that already had insulin dysregulation. However, this idea does not align with the fact that horses with PPID are 2.7 times more likely to have hyperinsulinaemia than healthy horses of the same age [214].

Clinical observations from veterinarians do indicate that horses with EMS may develop PPID at a younger age. In the absence of a clear conclusion, it is advisable to take a precautionary approach and actively work towards preventing EMS. In fact, it is a classic case of prevention being the better cure.

Horses affected by both EMS/ID and PPID exhibit more pronounced hyperinsulinaemia, increasing their susceptibility to laminitis compared to horses with either condition alone. As it currently stands, PPID-affected horses without EMS/ID do not necessarily display reduced insulin sensitivity [204].

A 2017 study even concluded that neither increased nor decreased dopaminergic activity, long- or short-term, had any impact on insulin production or insulin sensitivity in both insulin-resistant and insulin-sensitive horses [167].

Insulin sensitivity decreases by definition in older horses [79]. Given that PPID primarily affects older horses, we should also consider this as a partial explanation for overall insulin resistance. In fact, we cannot rule out the possibility that the combination of hyperinsulinaemia and PPID in horses aged over 15 is not related at all.

LAMINITIS

Severe laminitis is the most devastating manifestation of PPID. The prognosis is usually poor. The enduring, recurring intense pain associated with laminitis and the associated hoof abscesses (see sidebar on page 50), are the primary reasons most horse owners choose to opt for euthanasia.

Thankfully, not all equines affected by PPID develop laminitis. According to the aforementioned 2018 literature review, only 48.9% of them exhibit laminitis as a clinical manifestation [102]. Including cases of subclinical laminitis in the statistics would increase this percentage.

> **SUBCLINICAL**
> Early stage of a condition,
> in which no recognisable
> or observable clinical signs
> are evident.

An Australian study found that three out of four laminitic horses with PPID had insulin dysregulation too [131]. In another study, all horses with both PPID and laminitis also had hyper-insulinaemia [163]. The sample size in this study, however, was significantly smaller than that in the Australian study, with 16 horses compared to 274.

In contrast to acute laminitis, where a horse suddenly cannot move and is in obvious pain, laminitis in PPID-affected horses can be quite inconspicuous. A horse may display only minor hoof sensitivity or a shortened stride, which are also signs that could be attributed to arthritis or other age-related issues.

Clinical signs of laminitis may even go completely unnoticed at first in horses with PPID. This is because more beta-endorphin is produced. The horse's pain threshold increases as a result [117], with endorphins acting as pain suppressants. In the case of PPID, the effect appears to be as much as six times higher [105].

Because horses with PPID with incipient laminitis experience less pain, they may overload the damaged hoof tissue, consequently further increasing the damage [197].

In a 2019 study, 76% of PPID-afflicted horses were found to have laminitis. Their owners had only noticed this in 37% of cases [13].

Inexplicable laminitis and 15 years of age or older > always test for PPID (as soon as the laminitis is over) and insulin dysregulation. The same applies to horses that do get laminitis at the end of autumn, as opposed to during spring.

In some horses, laminitis is the only manifestation of PPID. Because of this, not every vet immediately thinks of PPID, particularly in the case of younger horses [126].

The side bar on page 69 tells you how to recognise laminitis. At the slightest suspicion, contact your vet and call your hoof care provider.

Let us now delve deeper into laminitis. If you want to gain a comprehensive understanding of this nasty disease, consider reading the book 'Laminitis : understanding, cure, prevention' (ISBN 978-94-93034-09-9).

ANATOMY OF THE HOOF

First, let's see how the hoof is composed *. If we look at the hoof from the outside, we see the hoof capsule. This fits around the so-called internal foot like a shoe. The hoof capsule consists of the hoof wall, the white line, the sole, the frog and the heel bulbs. The internal foot is made up of bones, tendons and ligaments, cartilage, connective tissue, skin, blood vessels, and nerves.

BONES AND TENDONS

The coffin bone is the lower bone in the hoof capsule. Together with the short pastern bone and the navicular bone, it forms the coffin joint (or distal interphalangeal joint). The deep digital flexor tendon runs over the navicular bone. This tendon is attached to the bottom of the coffin bone. On the other side, it is connected to the deep flexor muscle. The pull of the flexor muscle is transferred to the coffin bone through the tendon. The muscle and tendon enable the horse to flex the foot backwards. The extensor tendon connects the extensor muscle to the front of the coffin bone. This muscle and tendon enable the horse to stretch the foot forward.

HOOF CARTILAGES

The hoof cartilage, also referred to as collateral cartilage, are found at the back of the hoof and can be felt next to the bulb groove just above the level of the coronary band. At the bottom it merges into the digital cushion. This is connective tissue that acts as a shock absorber between the sole and the frog on one side and the tendons, bones, joints and hoof cartilage on the other.

UNDERSIDE OF THE HOOF

At the bottom of the hoof are the frog, the sole, the white line and the part of the hoof wall that touches the ground. The frog provides grip to the surface, contributes to shock absorption and plays an important role in the hoof mechanism, which involves the alternate expansion and contraction of the hoof when loaded and unloaded in motion. At its centre is the central groove (or central sulcus). A healthy central groove is wide and shallow.

The area between the frog and the hoof wall is called the sole. The horny tissue of the sole is firm and flexible. It provides protection to the coffin bone. A healthy sole is somewhat concave. The hollow shape contributes to the hoof mechanism and thus to good blood flow and shock absorption. The hoof wall and the sole are connected by the white line. Despite its name, it looks yellowish. A healthy white line is about two millimetres (0.8 inches) wide.

---

* See also the images on the next page

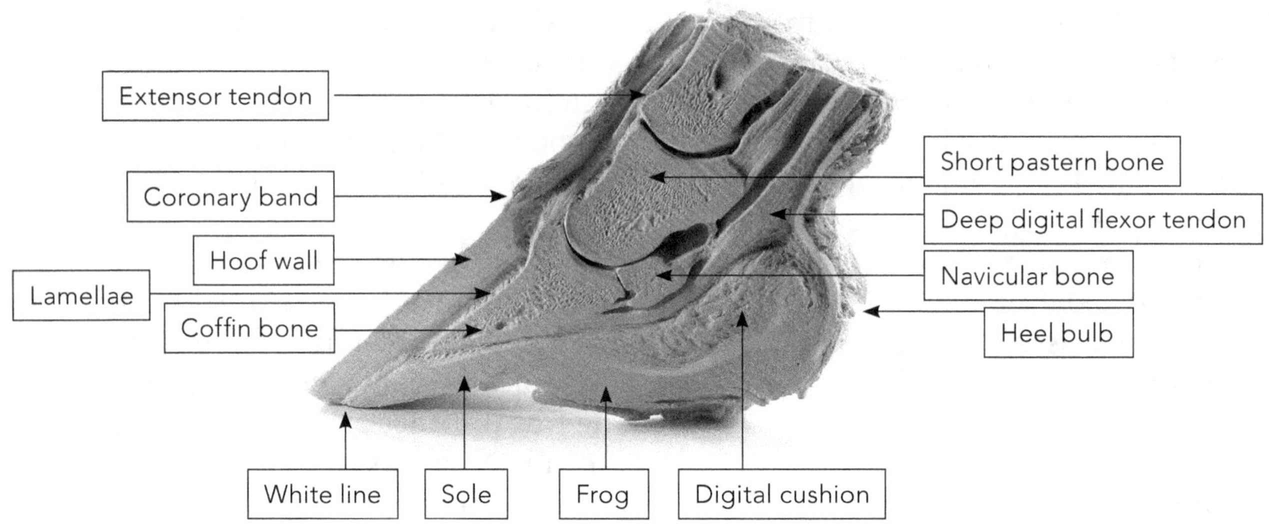

(plaster cast and photo: Christoph von Horst)

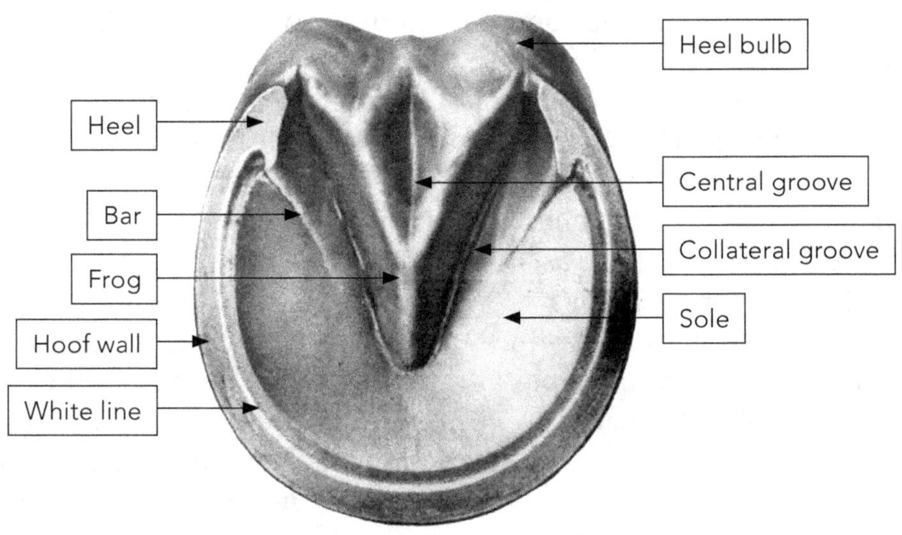

(illustration: W. Ellenberger)

HOOF WALL

The hoof wall is a thick horny layer that protects the vulnerable tissues inside the hoof and gives the hoof its strength. It is not intended to support the full body weight of the horse. The front part of the hoof wall is called the toe. If we compare the hoof with a clock, the toe is the part between 10 and 2 o'clock.

The back part of the hoof wall is called the heel. Each hoof wall has two heels. From there, the hoof wall bends back into the hoof. These specific parts are called the bars. They run parallel to the collateral grooves. The heel bulbs are located where the heels merge into the bulb groove.

LAMELLAR CONNECTION

The hoof wall is attached to the internal foot by a smart construction: the lamellar connection. This plays an important role in laminitis. That is why we will take a good look at it here. The entire internal foot is covered with hoof dermis. This is a tendon-like tissue full of blood vessels and nerves. The part of the dermis that surrounds the coffin bone and the hoof cartilages is called the wall dermis. The wall dermis is covered with approximately 600 thin strips of skin tissue: the dermal lamellae.

There are just as many epidermal lamellae (lamellar horn) on the inside of the hoof wall. The dermal and epidermal lamellae interlock like a kind of Velcro. To this end, they are covered with secondary lamellae. In between is a wafer-thin connective tissue membrane that attaches them to each other. This membrane is called the basement membrane. It is regarded as the most important connection in the structure of the hoof. It contains proteins that ensure the connection with the horn cells of the hoof wall. These are called hemidesmosomes. The lamellar connection consists of the two types of lamellae and the basement membrane together.

DESCRIPTION

A horse has laminitis if the lamellar connection is damaged to such an extent that the dermal and the epidermal lamellae are no longer held together. The connection between the hoof wall and the coffin bone breaks down. The coffin now starts to move within the hoof capsule. It will rotate and, in more severe cases, may sink vertically (sinker) or break through the sole (sole perforation).

CAUSES

Laminitis can be classified into three main types based on its primary causes. In the case of PPID, it falls under endocrinopathic laminitis, which is associated with hormonal problems. The other two types are SIRS-related laminitis, associated with systemic inflammatory response (also called sepsis-related laminitis), and traumatic laminitis, which is often referred to as supporting limb laminitis or road founder.

ABSCESSES AND LAMINITIS

Hoof abscesses can have different causes. In laminitis, we mainly see aseptic abscesses. They appear at the coronary band, in the white line, or above the hoof bulbs, typically one to two months after the onset of the laminitis. Aseptic means that the abscess was not caused by pathogens, such as bacteria.

Blood flow to the hoof is reduced in laminitis, caused in part by fluid build-up (oedema). Consequently, dead tissue and accumulated blood are not properly removed resulting in an aseptic hoof abscess. In the case of coffin bone rotation or a sinker, there will be pressure from the bone on the sole from within, causing additional tissue to die off, thereby further increasing the risk of an abscess developing.

As the abscess grows, the pressure on the surrounding tissues increases, as does the pain. In addition, septic abscesses can develop as bacteria enter the hoof through damaged tissue or the sole.

Because horses with PPID have lowered immunity, they are more prone to hoof abscesses, both septic and aseptic.

ENDOCRINOPATHIC LAMINITIS
Laminitis that occurs due to hormonal issues.

SIRS-RELATED LAMINITIS
Laminitis that occurs due to toxins in the bloodstream.

TRAUMATIC LAMINITIS
Laminitis that occurs due to heavy, prolonged, repetitive, or improper loading of the hooves on a hard surface.

In a Finnish study, nearly 90% of laminitis cases in horses that first presented with this issue at a veterinary university clinic, were attributed to endocrinopathic causes. Among this group, one in three had PPID [36].

CORTISOL OR EMS/INSULIN DYSREGULATION?

Veterinary science has not fully clarified the precise relationship between PPID and laminitis. Initially, it was believed that the fluctuations of cortisol levels throughout the day played a role in this. The direct influence of cortisol on hoof tissue, specifically the lamellar connection, was considered the primary cause.

There has now been a reversa of that theory; we now assume that EMS/insulin dysregulation is the main culprit [156, 214, 101]. Laminitis is, therefore, considered a secondary clinical manifestation and is not directly caused by PPID. In fact, endocrinopathic laminitis is not significantly more frequently diagnosed in horses with PPID than in horses without PPID unless insulin dysregulation has been identified as a concomitant condition [197].

It has not even been definitively established whether insulin dysregulation is a result of PPID in these cases. It may be possible that both conditions co-occur [222]. Nonetheless, they can still negatively influence each other. The melanocortins, of which there is a constant excess in the bloodstream of horses with PPID, have adverse effects on horses with EMS/ID and endocrinopathic laminitis [45, 156].

EMS/INSULIN DYSREGULATION

We can now examine how EMS/ID leads to laminitis. From your reading so far, it is clear that insulin is the hormone responsible for making body cells uptake sugar from the bloodstream. In the case of insulin dysregulation, there is too much insulin in the blood (hyperinsulinaemia), and the cells do not respond properly to insulin (insulin resistance). This results in inadequate sugar uptake, leading to elevated blood sugar levels (hyperglycaemia).

HYPERGLYCAEMIA

To start with the latter, hyperglycaemia contributes to laminitis through two mechanisms. Firstly, the excess sugar leads to the disruption of hemidesmosomes on the basement membrane. This results in the breakdown of the membrane's connection with the horn cells of the hoof wall.

Secondly, hyperglycaemia leads to the damage, constriction and clogging of capillaries in the hoof dermis. This, in turn, reduces blood flow to this tissue, including the basement membrane. As a consequence, the supply of oxygenated blood rich in nutrients, hormones and enzymes is compromised, as is the removal of oxygen-depleted (or carbon dioxide-rich) blood and waste products. This gradual deterioration affects the dermis, the dermal lamellae on it and the basement membrane, ultimately resulting in laminitis.

INSULIN

Insulin itself also plays a role in the development of laminitis. This is because insulin is involved in regulating blood vessel dilation and constriction. In a condition known as vascular insulin resistance, the vasodilatory effects of insulin are compromised, leading to blood vessel constriction [142]. This results in elevated blood pressure and reduced blood flow to the hoof tissue. Consequently, oxygen deficiency in the hoof tissue may occur, leading to cell death and an increased risk of laminitis.

Another consequence of excessive insulin in the bloodstream is the damage to the layer of cells lining the interior of blood vessels, known as the endothelium. This damage exacerbates capillary impairment.

IGF-1

Insulin-like growth factor 1 (IGF-1) is a hormone responsible for promoting the growth of cells and tissues. As the name implies, IGF-1 resembles insulin. Both have their own receptors within the body. In cases of hyperinsulinaemia, some of the insulin surplus will bind to IGF-1 receptors, which are notably abundant on the dermal lamellae.

The IGF-1 receptors respond to insulin as if it were IGF-1, prompting a growth stimulus. Consequently, dermal cells start multiplying and stay alive longer. This results in the secondary dermal lamellae becoming longer and narrower, thereby weakening their connection with the secondary epidermal lamellae [101, 163, 209]. This brings the horse another step closer to developing laminitis.

The aspects of endocrinopathic laminitis outlined here do not inherently induce pain [36]. Consequently, this type of laminitis often remains subclinical, going unnoticed. However, a vigilant hoof care provider or veterinarian can detect distinctive abnormalities in the hoof capsule, such as a stretched white line, disrupted growth rings and flares. Red spots in the hoof wall and sole are also a tell-tale sign. In all these instances, laminitis is, by definition, no longer considered subclinical as the features have become visibly apparent.

CORTISOL AND INSULIN

Cortisol may still play a role, given its inhibitory effect on insulin [237]. This effect is probably not substantial, as PPID-afflicted horses without clinical laminitis would otherwise have subclinical laminitis more often. However, a 2016 study found that these horses had no damage to lamellar tissue [163].

Apart from that, it is important to recognise that the pain associated with laminitis and other clinical signs of PPID leads to surges in cortisol levels. Cortisol has a vasoconstrictive effect, contributes to a rise in blood sugar levels and is associated with the development and worsening of insulin resistance. It can also play a role in the breakdown of hemidesmosomes in the basement membrane.

MELANOCORTINS

During spring, when the grass is full of fast sugars (see sidebar 'Sugar types' on page 125), there is an increase in laminitis cases among all horses, including those with PPID. However, the insulin peak in the bloodstream of grazing horses with PPID appears to be lower than during the seasonal rise in autumn [14]. This supports the idea that the body's insulin response is stronger under the influence of melanocortins. Yet, increased food intake in autumn may also be a contributing factor.

It is important to note that the sugar content in grass also rises in autumn. In summary, exercise caution with your PPID-affected horse in both spring and autumn, with heightened vigilance in autumn. Spring poses a greater risk for horses with both PPID and EMS/ID compared to those with PPID alone.

CLIP

A specific aspect of PPID is the melanocortin CLIP. Overproduction of this hormone in rats leads to heightened insulin production by the pancreas, subsequently contributing to insulin dysregulation [106, 156]. It has been theorised that a similar mechanism might occur in horses. This would then be of particular concern in horses with an existing genetic predisposition to insulin dysregulation, as the increased amount of CLIP then generates a heightened risk factor.

ALPHA-MSH

Alpha-MSH is also being looked at as a potential causative factor. Elevated levels of alpha-MSH are associated with fat storage [37]. Fat tissue acts as an endocrine gland, releasing adipokines, many of which reduce insulin sensitivity, induce vasoconstriction, and damage blood vessels. Three properties that can negatively contribute to the development of laminitis.

ESC

During the seasonal rise in ACTH and alpha-MSH, we also see an increase in the incidence of laminitis. During this period, particularly in September, horses grazing on pasture exhibit elevated blood glucose and insulin levels, which can be attributed to the higher levels of ethanol-soluble carbohydrates (ESC) in autumn grass. Conversely, horses kept in stables tend to demonstrate minimal to no hyperinsulinaemia during this time, provided their diet is as low in sugars as possible, of course.

SEASONAL RISE

Increase in ACTH and the derived melanocortins alpha-MSH and CLIP from mid-July to mid-November, peaking in September-October. Beta-endorphin probably also has this rise.

ESC

Ethanol-soluble carbohydrates. Single and double sugars, such as glucose, fructose and sucrose.

HYPERLIPIDAEMIA, HYPERTRIGLYCERIDAEMIA

Hyperlipidaemia is the presence of elevated fat concentrations in the blood, primarily involving a certain type of fat called triglycerides. So, it would be more accurate to refer to it as hypertriglyceridaemia. However, for the sake of readability, we will continue to use the term hyperlipidaemia, except in these specific paragraphs.

Hypertriglyceridaemia can lower insulin sensitivity and is a characteristic of EMS [107]. It can trigger blood vessel constriction in the hooves, resulting in decreased blood flow and subsequent deterioration of hoof tissue, encompassing the hoof dermis, dermal lamellae and basement membrane. Laminitis can strike or worsen now.

Hyperlipidaemia is more prevalent in ponies, donkeys and miniature horses compared to standard-sized horses. In donkeys, this is because they develop a loss of appetite (anorexia) in response to pain stemming from complications of PPID, notably laminitis. Anorexia may lead to the onset of hyperlipidaemia [199].

Hyperlipidaemia is associated with various factors, including stress, sudden food deprivation (overly strict diets!), prolonged consumption of high-sugar feeds, and obesity [107].

ADRENAL ENLARGEMENT

Adrenal gland enlargement, or adrenomegaly, is present in approximately 20% of horses with PPID [117, 130, 203]. This condition results from abnormal cell division (hyperplasia) and cell enlargement (hypertrophy), triggered by excessive ACTH levels in the bloodstream and the six-fold increased action of ACTH under the influence of alpha-MSH and beta-endorphin [15].

Adrenal enlargement results in heightened cortisol production. Yet, chronic ACTH-dependent hypercortisolaemia is infrequently observed in horses with PPID [59, 229].

ORGAN DAMAGE

The lungs, kidneys, liver, heart, thyroid, and adrenal glands can also be impacted in horses with PPID, a fact that remains relatively unfamiliar among veterinarians. Moreover, diagnosing such issues can be exceedingly challenging when the vet is attending at a client's premises.

To illustrate, during autopsies, it was discovered that nearly 75% of the 26 horses with PPID had swollen liver cells. In contrast, the control group exhibited a percentage just slightly exceeding 15% [130].

EARLY AND ADVANCED STAGES

Clinical signs can be classified according to when they appear during the disease progression, providing insight into whether PPID is in its early or advanced stage.

EARLY STAGE

- Behavioural changes, particularly apathy
- Partial, regional hypertrichosis, delayed shedding and coat discolouration
- Reduced muscle mass on shoulders and back
- Hyper- or hypohidrosis
- Infertility
- Adiposity
- Laminitis
- Tendinitis/desmitis

ADVANCED STAGE

- Advanced forms of the early clinical signs
- Behavioural changes, especially exercise intolerance
- Generalised hypertrichosis, loss of hair, coat shedding
- Advanced muscle atrophy extending to withers and glutes
- 'Pot belly', due to muscle atrophy
- Polyuria/polydipsia
- Recurrent infections and abscesses, corneal ulcers
- Increased mammary gland secretion (milky discharge)
- Tendon and suspensory ligament laxity
- Neurological issues

SUMMARY

PPID differs from Cushing's disease or syndrome. In PPID, there is a disruption in the function of the intermediate lobe of the pituitary gland, leading to a cascade of hormonal imbalances. The pituitary gland's dysregulation is attributed to a dopamine deficiency resulting from neurodegeneration. This may lead to the swelling of the intermediate lobe and the development of glandular tissue tumours.

One common manifestation of PPID is cortisol dysregulation, where various cortisol-related processes become disrupted. However, the total amount of cortisol in the blood typically remains within the normal range. This hormonal dysregulation, coupled with the pressure exerted by the enlarged pituitary gland on brain tissue, can give rise to a diverse range of clinical signs.

The most prevalent signs include excessive hair growth, laminitis and muscle loss. Additionally, a significant proportion of horses with PPID are also affected by the metabolic disorder EMS, where insulin dysregulation plays a central role and is considered the primary cause of laminitis in these horses.

CAUSES

The slow development of PPID makes identifying its causes difficult. Clinical signs emerge only after a long period of time – sometimes years. Moreover, the disease cannot be induced experimentally. As a result, we still do not know for sure what causes PPID.

The explanation for the breakdown of dopamine-producing nerves running from the hypothalamus to the pituitary gland is mainly considered to be due to an abundance of free radicals in the pituitary gland and the resulting oxidative stress. Two other partial causes being studied are mitochondrial dysfunction and in the functionality of the protein alpha-synuclein.

FREE RADICALS AND OXIDATIVE STRESS

Oxidative stress is essentially an imbalance between free radicals (oxidants) and antioxidants, where the action of free radicals surpasses the ability of antioxidants to neutralise them, resulting in cell and, consequently, tissue damage.

Free radicals are by-products of normal metabolism. They are molecules that lack an electron (negatively charged particle). As a result, they become unstable. In an effort to regain stability, they bind to an electron of an oxygen molecule from one of the surrounding cells.

In a healthy metabolism, this is not a problem. In fact, some free radicals have an important function in combating viruses and inflammation. However, the scenario changes if free radicals are produced as a result of inflammation, a worm infestation, medication, residues of pesticides or fertilisers on food, contaminated water (heavy metals), excessive or insufficient exercise, stress, hyperglycaemia, obesity, or adiposity.

This creates an excess of free radicals in the body and too many bond with oxygen molecules from healthy tissue cells, consequently, causing the latter to become damaged. This cycle continues and if the body can not intervene, a chain reaction ensues.

In studies using laboratory animals to investigate Parkinson's disease, oxidative stress and neurodegeneration were observed following pesticide exposure. A 2019 systematic literature review found that occupational exposure to pesticides was at least 50% more likely to cause neurodegenerative disease [183].

LOCAL OXIDATIVE STRESS

It is notable that systemic oxidative stress – i.e., stress caused throughout the body – is only seen to a limited extent in horses with PPID [18, 243]. However, local oxidative stress is evident in the intermediate lobe of the pituitary gland, also known as pars intermedia oxidative stress [191].

Our current assumption is that local oxidative stress is the primary cause of PPID, potentially explaining nerve degradation. Notably, dopaminergic nerve cells are highly sensitive to oxidative stress [177].

From human medicine, we know that there is a link between oxidative stress and neurodegenerative diseases, such as Alzheimer's disease, Parkinson's disease and multiple sclerosis.

3-NITROTYROSINE

In 2005, a widely referenced study discovered a 16-fold rise in the enzyme 3-nitrotyrosine (3-N) within the dopamine-producing nerve endings in the hypothalamus of horses with PPID, in contrast to healthy horses [177]. 3-N serves as a biomarker signalling the presence of oxidative stress.

> ### BIOMARKER
> A measurable indication of a biological state or condition.

At higher concentrations of 3-N, the amount of the antioxidant glutathione peroxidase also increases, suggesting oxidative stress as a significant causative factor in PPID. We also see elevated concentrations of this substance in people with the aforementioned neurodegenerative disorders [1].

In healthy, older horses, the concentration of 3-N in the intermediate lobe also increases. This may mean that oxidative stress of this part of the pituitary gland may be a normal feature of ageing.

LIPOFUSCIN

Another indication of oxidative stress as a cause was found in 2009, when research revealed abundant lipofuscin in nerves. Lipofuscin can be considered as oxidised cellular debris [130].

IL-8

On page 35 under 'Infections and inflammation', we have already covered interleukin-8 (IL-8). This pro-inflammatory protein is elevated in PPID-affected horses, potentially contributing to chronic low-grade inflammation, oxidative stress, and nerve breakdown [78].

ANTIOXIDANT CAPACITY AND SUSCEPTIBILITY TO DAMAGE

The occurrence of free radicals is just one part of the problem. Leading on from there is the body's inability to neutralise them. Inadequate antioxidant capacity can stem from impaired activity of antioxidant enzymes and from a lack of antioxidants in the diet. Furthermore, in some horses, nerves in general may be more susceptible to damage from free radicals.

MnSOD

Manganese Superoxide Dismutase (MnSOD) is an antioxidant enzyme that shields body cells from free radical damage. In aged horses, the activity of MnSOD in the intermediate lobe of the pituitary gland decreases. This might partially explain oxidative stress and nerve degradation [240]. Similar to the rise in 3-N, the decline in MnSOD would be a normal feature of aging. Some scientists propose that ageing is even the main cause of PPID, partly because dopaminergic nerve numbers decrease even in older horses without PPID.

OTHER CAUSES OF IMPAIRED ENZYMATIC ACTIVITY

Impaired enzyme activity can result from various factors, including genetics, stress, insufficient protein in the diet, or deficiencies in vitamins (A, D, E, a.o.) and minerals (selenium, copper, chromium, zinc, a.o.). Even a severe worm infestation negatively affects antioxidant formation.

It is beyond the scope of this book to discuss all of these aspects. In essence, we can say that the healthier and more akin to its natural environment that you can keep your horse, the better this will be for the body's capacity to deal with antioxidants. This is of paramount importance, as the problem may well worsen if the causes are not reduced or eliminated.

TOXINS

Previously, we touched on fertilisers and pesticides as toxins causing excess free radicals and oxidative stress. Discussing all toxins burdening the equine body would make this book quite thick, so we will not do that. However, we will briefly categorise and provide a few examples.

The following types of toxins can be distinguished: bacterial and non-bacterial toxins, poisonous plants, pollution, and chemical toxins. Note, this list is not meant to be exhaustive.

BACTERIAL TOXINS

A notorious cause of bacterial toxins in the horse's body, is consuming food with lots of fast carbohydrates, like grass containing high quantities of sugar. When there is more sugar than the small intestine can digest, these sugars reach the large intestine, causing acidification. Consequently, bacterial die-off occurs in the gut, releasing toxins into the bloodstream.

Bacterial toxins in the bloodstream can also arise from influenza, colic, or inflammation, such as lung, eye, or uterine infections. As mentioned on page 40, EOTRH can also be a source.

NON-BACTERIAL TOXINS

Non-bacterial toxins encompass mycotoxins, which are given off by moulds, fungi and yeasts. Mouldy hay or grass silage can be considered as potential sources of these toxins.

POISONOUS PLANTS

At the top of the list of plants poisonous to horses are privet, yew, boxwood, maple and Jacob's wort, followed by oak (the unripe, green acorns and the leaves are toxic), beech (the nuts), laburnum, false acacia and rhododendron. However the full list is much longer than we can cover here.

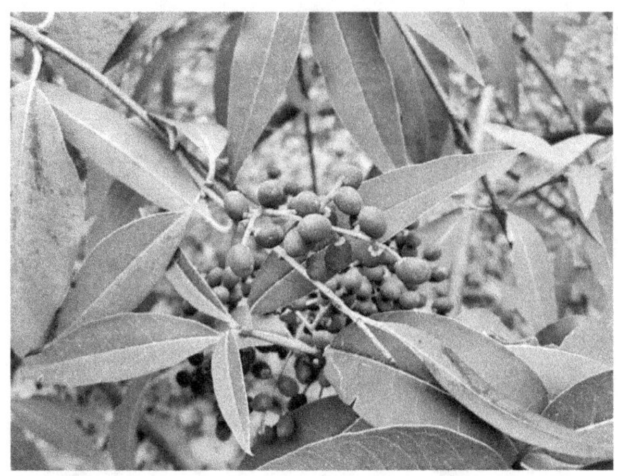

Privet is highly toxic to horses
(*photo: Michael Kesl*)

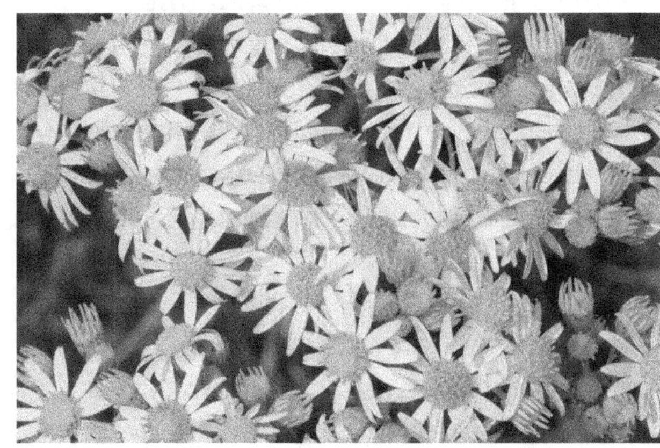

Jacob's wort
(*photo: Vladimír Motyčka*)

During conditions such as prolonged drought, heavy snowfall, or periods of restricted food intake like grazing restrictions, horses are more likely to eat any available food, increasing the risk of consuming poisonous plants.

In autumn, when trees and shrubs drop their seeds and leaves, the likelihood of horses ingesting toxins through this route is also higher.

> *Horses that are low in the hierarchy, such as old or those weakened by PPID, may be chased away from food by higher-ranking grazing companions. This could lead them to eat from poisonous trees and shrubs.*

Certain poisonous plants taste bitter when fresh but turn sweeter as they dry. When pulling weeds, never leave them in the pasture. Also, always check the hay before offering it and remove any dried plants that you don't recognise.

Pollution and chemical toxins

These toxins include contaminated water, pesticides and undecomposed fertilisers.

Prolonged exposure to a glyphosate-based herbicide leads to dopaminergic nerve breakdown in a certain type of worm used widely in research on neurodegenerative diseases in humans [129]. This obviously does not tell us whether the same is true in horses.

Of course, acute PPID will not result from a horse nibbling on a poisonous plant or having an eye infection. A direct link between oxidative stress and PPID has not been proven for each toxin mentioned either. Nevertheless, it is worth checking the long-term toxins your horse encounters and eliminating them. If your horse already has PPID, this might help prevent the ailment from worsening.

Stress

In human medicine, researchers are exploring the connection between chronic stress and an increase in specific pro-inflammatory proteins. This could potentially contribute negatively to low-grade inflammation and, consequently, oxidative stress [24, 153]. Whether this mechanism operates similarly in horses, is as yen unclear.

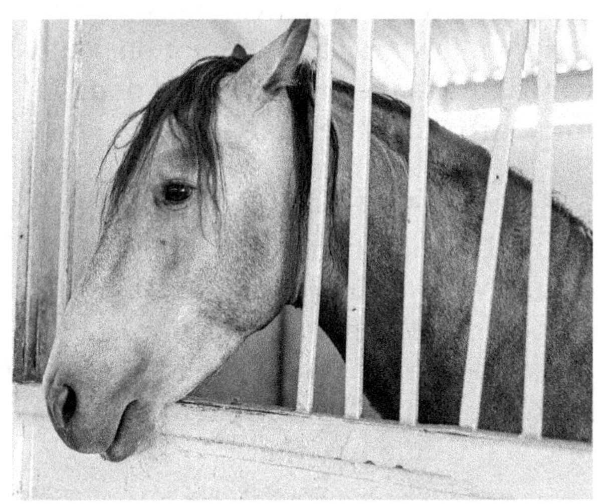

Chronic stress behind the bars
(photo: Rodnae productions)

EMS AND CHRONIC LOW-GRADE INFLAMMATION

Adipose tissue acts like a gland, releasing substances with immune system functions, called adipokines. See page 44 in relation to laminitis.

Adipokines act as messengers for the immune system. Some of them promote inflammation primarily because the body uses inflammation as part of its arsenal to fight off bacteria, viruses and other foreign invaders.

An elevation in pro-inflammatory adipokines contributes to the emergence of low-grade inflammation, meaning the body is in a constant state of inflammation. The immune system is continuously active, but at such low levels that no classical inflammatory signs occur. We now know that low-grade inflammation is associated with the development of PPID and the oxidative stress resulting from low-grade inflammation could contribute to the breakdown of dopamine-producing nerves.

Leptin, interleukin-6 (IL-6) and tumour necrosis factor-alpha (TNF-alpha) are examples of such pro-inflammatory adipokines. Elevated production of these adipokines leads to an increase in free radicals and hence chronic, low-grade inflammation [62, 152, 156].

Elevated levels of leptin and IL-6 are associated with impaired cortisol binding [62]. This would cause more free cortisol in the blood. On page 24 you have read why science is looking at this with interest.

MITOCHONDRIAL DYSFUNCTION

A second possible partial cause is mitochondrial dysfunction (disruption of the normal function of mitochondria). A mitochondrion is a cellular organelle that plays a crucial role in cell metabolism, particularly in energy conversion. A common metaphor for the mitochondrion in biology textbooks is 'the powerhouse of the cell'. Mitochondria are found in the vast majority of the body's cells and thus also in the cells of the dopamine-producing nerves.

From human medicine, we know that something can go wrong in the process of energy conversion, causing an overproduction of free radicals [173]. As previously covered, free radicals will attempt to grab electrons from surrounding cells, in this case, this includes electrons from the DNA of the mitochondria themselves. As a result, the DNA mutates. The nerve cell can no longer function properly; among other things, its energy supply is compromised. This, in turn, can lead to cell death and death of the nerve.

As mitochondrial dysfunction progresses, impending cell death will come closer and closer at an increasingly rapid pace. This is because cell metabolism becomes more and more unbalanced, which in turn leads to a growing accumulation of free radicals.

Mitochondrial dysfunction is a hallmark of ageing and of chronic diseases in general.

ALPHA-SYNUCLEIN

Alpha-synuclein is a protein found mainly in the brain, particularly in the ends of nerve cells that release neurotransmitters. The exact physiological function of alpha-synuclein is not known, but it may help regulate dopamine release.

In people with Parkinson's disease, we see that alpha-synuclein is misfolded, accumulates and clumps together in long fibres, damaging nerve cells [149].

PROTEIN AGGREGATION

Protein folding is the process by which a protein attains its functional and biologically active three-dimensional structure. The accumulation and clumping together of misfolded proteins is called protein aggregation.

In equines affected by PPID, greater amounts of alpha-synuclein are found in the intermediate lobe of the pituitary than in healthy horses of the same age. This, as in Parkinson's disease, would potentially lead to the breakdown of dopamine-producing nerves [149, 177]. A significant portion of the alpha-synuclein is misfolded [118].

Oxidative stress and antioxidant deficiency, according to 2005 research, combined together could create conditions conducive to protein aggregation [243]. The question is as yet open ended as to whether fibrous protein accumulations cause nerve degradation or result from it.

Cells have mechanisms that can refold or break down protein aggregates. In older horses, these control mechanisms might not function as efficiently [185].

The intriguing parallels highlighted here have led human medicine to look at whether PPID-afflicted horses could serve as laboratory animals for studying Parkinson's disease and other neurodegenerative conditions.

SUMMARY

The precise cause of PPID is not yet known. It is highly likely that nerve break-down is mainly due to an imbalance between free radicals (oxidants) and antioxidants in the pituitary gland. We call this oxidative stress. The balance is disrupted by an excess of free radicals entering or forming in the body, coupled with the body's inability to neutralise them effectively.

Another potential cause involves a malfunction in a specific component of nerve cells (mitochondria). Finally, abnormalities in specific proteins within dopamine-producing nerve cells could contribute to the issue.

DIAGNOSIS

Treating without knowing exactly what you are treating or to what extent your horse is suffering from an ailment is fruitless. Even if you think you know for sure that your horse has PPID, you will have to have the diagnosis made by a veterinarian. Besides the anamnesis and clinical examination, blood tests to either identify or rule out both PPID and EMS play an important role in the diagnosis.

PPID is a slowly progressive and incurable disease with many fluctuations in hormone production and all kinds of overlapping, mutually reinforcing and counteracting aspects and processes. Early diagnosis of PPID is difficult as a result.

Horse owners often mistakenly regard the early manifestations of PPID as common signs of ageing. They usually consult a vet only when secondary conditions like laminitis occur or advanced signs become apparent (see sidebar 'Early and advanced stages' on page 55).

Subclinical PPID might be present for months to years before the first clinical signs emerge. After all, the internal breakdown of nerves is invisible from the outside.

LAMINITIS

This nasty disease is mainly due to EMS/insulin dysregulation. While PPID and EMS/ID can occur simultaneously, they should be diagnosed separately. Thankfully, veterinarians nowadays more routinely test for hormonal abnormalities in laminitis than in the past.

The pain associated with laminitis can be mitigated by the high levels of beta-endorphin. This means that there is less pain than you would expect given the severity of the laminitis. This is another reason why we often do not notice laminitis until too late. If, due to the higher pain threshold, the horse additionally overstrains the already compromised hoof tissue, the situation worsens.

DIAGNOSIS

All this often stands in the way of timely intervention. This is unfortunate, as early recognition of the disease greatly improves the horse's quality of life and life expectancy making a difference to the horse owner's remaining possibilities to use their horse.

PPID must be diagnosed based on anamnesis, clinical examination and blood tests in tandem. It is not feasible to confirm or rule out PPID based solely on blood tests or the clinical signs alone as the most common of these may also have a cause other than PPID.

Equally when blood test results clearly point in the direction of PPID, while the clinical picture is good, veterinarians should revaluate their clinical examination. They may be overlooking something, because, for example, the most common signs were not convincingly present. It will not be the first time that PPID is not recognised because the horse does not have a curly coat.

Medical imaging actually takes place primarily in a scientific context, for example during post-mortem examinations (autopsy).

ANAMNESIS

The anamnesis is the mapping of the disease history through a medical history assessment. With a chronic, slow-developing disease such as PPID, where the cause is not yet known with absolute certainty, this assessment will mainly focus on the clinical signs and their severity in your horse.

Especially if your horse is laminitic as well, your veterinarian will ask you many questions to get as complete a picture as possible. Together with you, they aim to grasp all the factors that could have contributed to the complications.

In determining the prognosis, they will also need information. How old is your horse? What factors are promoting or hindering recovery from the complications? Any information you as an owner can provide holds significance. Do not hesitate to share your observations with the vet.

The anamnesis may cover the following points:
- Living conditions
  - How long has the horse been with you?
  - Nutrition. Is your horse eating well? What is its weight? Is it underweight or overweight and what causes this? Did your horse previously weigh more or less?

- How is it housed? What is your usual exercise schedule?
- Use of the horse
  - What are your expectations about the course of the disease and the future use of your horse?
- The vet will ask you if you have observed behavioural changes or exercise intolerance and if your horse drinks and urinates more than before.
- If your horse is in an advanced stage of PPID, there may also be neurological problems the vet could ask about.
- Veterinary history
  - Did the horse already have PPID when you got it?
  - Has there been a previous diagnosis of PPID or EMS/insulin dysregulation? What was it? Are there results of blood tests and treatment plans? Are there results of imaging studies, such as hoof X-rays, in the case of laminitis?
  - Is or was the horse on medication or supplements for PPID or its complications? Which ones, dosage, and effectiveness?
  - How does your horse shed after winter? Do you shave your horse and, if so, how often? Does it sweat a lot or quickly?
- Other treatment providers
  - Who is the hoof care provider? Is your horse shod, barefoot or does it have hoof boots? Since when?
- Is a nutritionist involved? Is there a dietary plan, and if not, what does your horse eat? How is its appetite?
- Do you have an equine dentist? How often do they visit, and when was the last time? What were their findings and actions?
- Is your horse up-to-date with its vaccinations and worming treatments?
- Has your horse been seen and treated by other specialists, related or unrelated to PPID? Are treatment plans available, and are they effective?

CLINICAL EXAMINATION

Clinical examination usually starts from establishing the presence of easily recognisable clinical signs. Here, the vet will make their own observations of what has been discussed in anamnesis, focusing on details that you, as the owner, may have overlooked or might not recognise.

Generalised (complete) hypertrichosis, a sign of advanced PPID, will be noticed immediately by the vet. Common signs like polyuria and polydipsia are also easily noticeable. This is why the vet inquired about your horse's drinking and urination during the anamnesis. Visible emaciation, decreased muscle mass on the back, and a pot belly are also easy to spot. The clinical examination also involves closely examining your horse's dental condition.

Endocrinopathic (or: hormone-related) laminitis goes undetected more often than SIRS-related laminitis due to its latent onset. Attention is therefore called for. The sidebar on the page opposite tells you how your vet (or yourself, of course) can recognise laminitis.

Again: inexplicable laminitis, especially in autumn, is often the first sign of PPID.

EMS/INSULIN DYSREGULATION

Since insulin dysregulation affects at least one in three horses with PPID and is a distinctive feature of EMS, your veterinarian will also search for signs of this hormonal abnormality in the clinical examination.

BODY CONDITION

To do so, they use the Body Condition Score (BCS) or Henneke's scale and the Cresty Neck Score (CNS). The BCS classifies a horse's body condition by examining fat distribution on specific parts and assigning a grade.

A score of one or two is for horses considered to be too lean, three and four are considered fair and good, and five and six signal concerns, especially for insulin-resistant horses, meaning they are tending towards obesity.

Donkeys are assessed with a modified BCS. What may be considered 'good' for horses is often deemed 'fat' for donkeys. Many donkey owners may not be aware that their donkey is overweight.

Another rating system, Henneke's scale, assigns points to fat distribution on specific body parts as well, averaging them. The scale ranges from one to nine, where one stands for emaciated and nine for extremely fat. For most horses, the optimal score is four, five or six.

The CNS is used to assess neck circumference and thus obesity. It uses a six-point scale where a result of four and above is considered unfavourable.

You can track your horse's BCS/Henneke and CNS in the log mentioned on page 27, but it is not infallible. Normal variations can occur due to factors like age, breed, season, and horse use. These systems serve as tools; your veterinarian or equine nutritionist can provide a broader perspective on the scores.

Continue on page 72

RECOGNISING LAMINITIS

In all three types of laminitis (endocrinopathic, SIRS-related, traumatic), similar clinical signs appear, such as increased hoof temperature, reluctance to move, leaning backward, and lethargic behaviour. With SIRS-related laminitis these signs present early in the disease, whereas in endocrinopathic laminitis, they are less common. The latter typically has a subtle onset, with the horse not always experiencing pain. This may be due to dysregulation of cortisol metabolism (see page 24). This is because corticosteroids have an analgesic effect. Also, unlike SIRS-related laminitis, it is less frequently accompanied by painful inflammation of the lamellar tissue. Consequently, this type of laminitis remains more often subclinical and therefore unnoticed. Early detection of endocrinopathic laminitis through abnormal hoof growth (disrupted growth rings, which are no longer parallel to the coronary band, a stretched white line, and a flaring hoof wall) or red spots in the hoof wall and sole (sole bruising), can therefore make a substantial difference to the prognosis. If you have an attentive and experienced hoof care provider and vet, you are already more likely to catch it in time. Regular and frequent visits from the hoof care provider are therefore also very important.

In particular, disrupted growth rings, resulting from shape change of the secondary epidermal lamellae (see page 49), are an important clue [189]. The formation of this growth anomaly typically spans around three months, often surpassing the owner's awareness of the presence of laminitis. These changes are usually – and thus sometimes wrongly – associated with previous or chronic laminitis.

If there is indeed pain, we see some or all of the following signs:

- Strong and rapid pulse (80-120 beats per minute)
- Muscle tremors and higher muscle tension
- Sweating (be careful not to confuse this with hyperhidrosis, as described on page 30)
- Dehydration
- Dilated pupils, excessive blood flow to the ocular mucosa
- Widened nostrils, ears stiffly turned backwards
- Rapid or irregular and erratic breathing (80-100 breaths per minute).
  Old horses tend to breathe faster than young ones. Take this into account.
- Increased body temperature (40-41 °C / 104-106 °F)
- Hot feet, pulsations
- Hoof abscesses
- Stiff or not wanting to move at all, difficulty with turns, more lame on a hard surface than on a soft one
- Laminitic stance (leaning backwards), shifting of weight, sometimes the feet are alternately lifted, lying down a lot.
- Irritability, anxiety, being withdrawn, sighing and moaning

To assess lameness, the veterinarian might employ the Obel grading system, which you will learn more about in the next sidebar.

The vet can often see his suspicion of laminitis confirmed using X-rays, even in the acute phase we are talking about here.

Once the coffin bone begins to rotate within the hoof capsule, the chronic phase has begun. Anomalies occur to the normal anatomy of the hoof, both visible changes on the outside and those that are only detectable through X-rays.

One of the better known of these is the lamellar wedge. As the coffin bone becomes loose and starts to tilt, a space is left between the coffin bone and the hoof wall in the toe region of the hoof. This space fills up with proliferating horny cells, old inflammatory blood, blood serum, necrotic (dead) hoof tissue and new inflammations, collectively called the lamellar wedge.

The rotating coffin bone pulls down the tissue from which the hoof wall grows. This will create a deep ring in the hoof wall, visible a few days after the onset of laminitis. It then grows downwards from the coronary band.

Flares are fanning out deformations of the hoof wall. They occur because the lamellar connection is not sufficiently capable of absorbing the long-term mechanical forces on the hoof wall.

Apart from these three easily recognisable characteristics of chronic laminitis, there is a wide range of problematic features that increase in severity as the disease advances. The book 'Laminitis : understanding, cure, prevention' discusses them in detail. Here we are limiting ourselves to noting that just about any part of the hoof can inflame, deform, loosen, break or die. The most prevalent complications will be discussed from page 143 onwards.

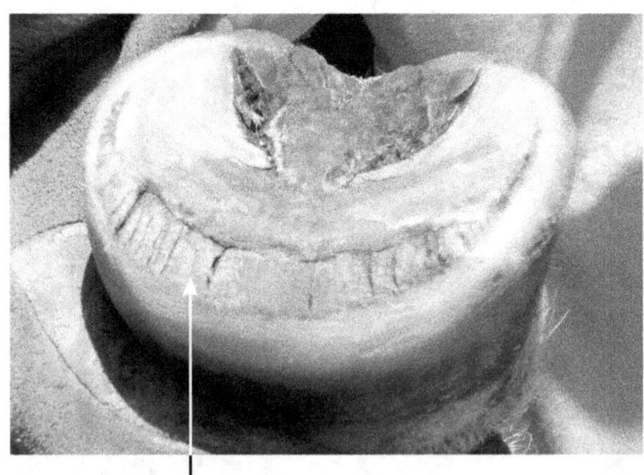

Lamellar wedge
(photo: Cynthia Cooper)

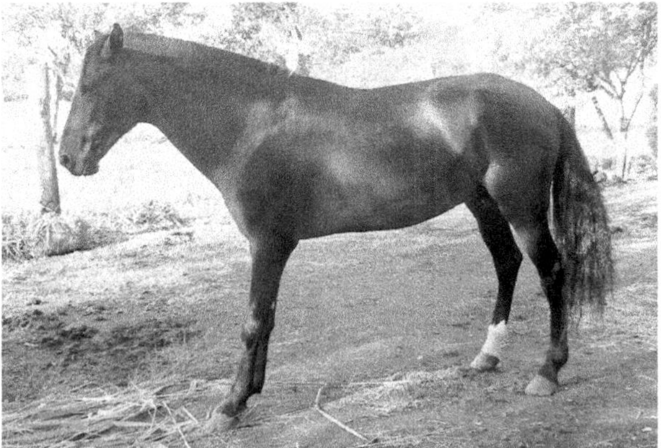

Laminitis stance
(photo: Advanced Equine Therapies)

THE MODIFIED OBEL METHOD

In 1948, Niles Obel created a grading system to classify the degree of lameness in laminitis. The scale runs from 0 to 4, with Obel 0 representing 'all movement is without problems' and Obel 4 representing 'horse refuses to move'. The higher the score, the more severe the lameness. Veterinarians and hoof care providers utilise this system to track healing progress. A horse that goes from Obel 4 to Obel 3 is on the path to recovery.

The system however, has limitations; primarily, it is not very accurate with only five categories, making it challenging to detect subtle changes in pain. Another major limitation of this system is that it is based on SIRS-related laminitis, whereas PPID-afflicted horses face endocrinopathic laminitis. In this form, the clinical manifestation of pain is often milder, it may start more insidiously or fall between two Obel classes. If it is between Obel 0 and 1, there is a risk that the laminitis will go unnoticed.

There was an urgency therefore, driven by the scientific community for the creation of a modified Obel scale to more accurately assess the severity of endocrinopathic laminitis. The solution, known as the modified Obel method or Meier method, is a rating system assigning points to clinical signs. The sum of these points provides a score on a scale of 0 to 12.

When employing this system, assessors frequently arrive at consistent outcomes upon re-assessment, and different assessors commonly agree on the same horse [175].

Currently, the modified Obel method is only used by scientific researchers in testing treatment and prevention methods. It would be beneficial if this method could be integrated into veterinary practices.

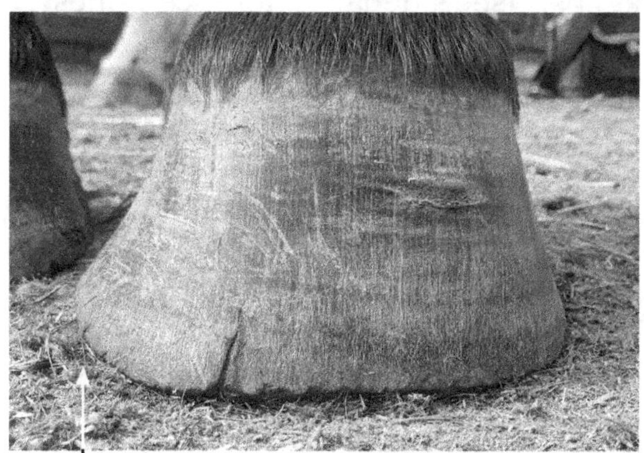

Flare

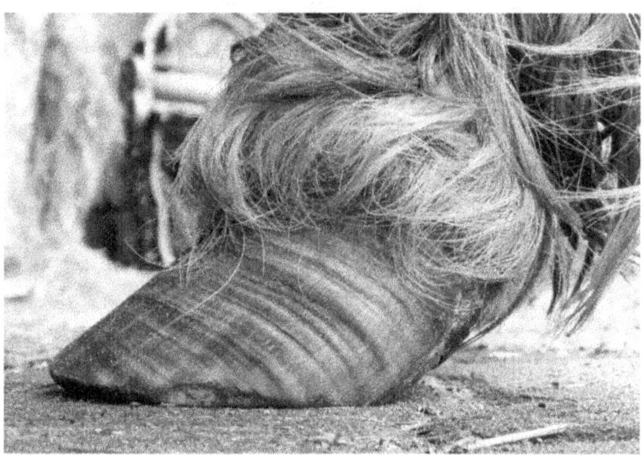

Laminitic rings

To identify signs of adiposity, the vet will check for fat accumulation above the eyes, in the sheath (in males) or udder (in mares), and trunk.

High blood pressure is also a manifestation of EMS, as are polyuria, polydipsia and apathy.

BLOOD TEST

Standard blood tests do not directly detect the presence of PPID, but can reveal secondary infections, which might prompt the vet to decide to look further for PPID.

Although mild anaemia and abnormalities in numbers of certain white blood cells are sometimes detected in PPID-afflicted equines, too little is known about how often this actually occurs. Therefore, they are not utilised as diagnostic criteria for PPID.

Elevated levels of liver enzymes are found in the blood in some PPID-affected horses, suggesting the possibility of corticosteroid-induced liver disease [117].

ENDOCRINOLOGICAL BLOOD TESTS

For less advanced cases, identifying subclinical and uncertain instances, and gauging treatment response, laboratory diagnostics – especially endocrinological blood tests – are important.

Confirmation of the disease through blood tests offers reassurance to horse owners hesitant about committing to lifelong medication.

Endocrinological blood tests without the presence of clinical signs are a moot point. The likelihood of a false-positive result is high (see sidebar on the opposite page). This is especially true in young horses with inconclusive clinical signs. This reinforces the need to combine blood testing with the clinical presentation to indicate PPID. However, there is something to be said for the fact that early intervention in subclinical cases may prevent a lot of misery in the future.

Recent research has focused on improving the interpretation of blood test results under different conditions. As a result, many more grey areas have developed making it more difficult to have a clear cut-off value to make a diagnosis (see sidebar 'Reference values' on the opposite page).

In the grey areas, hormone levels may be normal despite the presence of clinical signs or vice versa: elevated hormone levels with no clinical signs.

Re-testing during the peak of the seasonal rise in September-October is recommended. Employing a different test type could also provide more clarity.

If there are few or only mild clinical signs with normal hormone levels, the vet should look further into other possible causes for the abnormal clinical picture.

TYPES OF TESTS

Certain tests are suitable for in-home testing, while others are more effectively conducted at the clinic. The latter is preferred when blood needs to be drawn at specific intervals or when special materials are required for processing the blood sample.

There are basal tests and dynamic tests. Basal tests involve taking a single blood sample to assess the quantity of a particular substance, like a hormone, present in the blood. Dynamic tests, on the other hand, begin by analysing a blood sample to measure the levels of specific substances. This initial examination serves as the baseline measurement. Next, a substance is fed or injected into the horse. A second blood sample is collected after some time to observe the changes that have taken place under the influence of this substance.

For the tests discussed below, it is advisable to conduct testing at least once a year, but ideally twice a year. This allows monitoring of changes in the blood count and assessment of whether any adjustments to medication are necessary.

FALSE POSITIVES AND FALSE NEGATIVES

With a false positive result, a test wrongly shows that the horse is suffering from a particular ailment or has abnormalities in its blood count.

Conversely, with a false negative result, the situation is reversed: the horse has the disease or abnormal blood values, but the test fails to detect it.

Both scenarios are undesirable. A false positive result can mean the horse faces overtreatment; false negative means undertreatment. In the case of overtreatment, the horse needlessly undergoes potentially harmful treatments and medications, while in the case of undertreatment it does not receive the care it needs.

REFERENCE VALUES

In blood tests, we use reference values. These are two outer limits that define acceptable or normal outcomes, often referred to as normal values or lab values. The vast majority of healthy horses fall within those values.

If blood test results fall outside these values, whether higher or lower, the vet will see this as a reason to confirm their suspicions gathered from the anamnesis and clinical examination. When the result falls within the reference values, the vet can then proceed with their investigation, having potentially eliminated a diagnostic suspicion. Subsequent blood tests are often required to compare and contrast the results to the reference values, enabling the vet to make an informed analysis whether the horse is or is not suffering from the suspected illness or that is has begun to recover following treatment.

It is also encouraging if the results show that all the efforts you make to improve your horse's insulin sensitivity with exercise and dietary adjustments are paying off.

ACTH-TEST

This is a basal test that measures the amount of ACTH in the blood plasma. As explained on page 23, horses with PPID exhibit elevated ACTH levels. This is attributed to increased production from the precursor POMC. Additionally, the conversion into derived hormones lags behind this heightened production.

Assuming that ACTH generated in the intermediate lobe of the pituitary gland is biologically less potent than ACTH from the anterior lobe of a healthy pituitary, we encounter a constraint in ACTH testing. This is because the test indicates the presence of ACTH but does not provide information about its biological activity or its specific origin within the pituitary.

There are horses with high ACTH levels that do not have PPID. Do not fixate on the outcome of an ACTH test alone. The clinical presentation holds equal significance. You will find additional information later about factors that can lead to an increase in ACTH levels, besides PPID.

As the disease progresses, the test's reliability increases.

A meta-analysis of ten studies in 2020 found test sensitivity to be 68% and test specificity to be 86% [3]. The first percentage signifies how often the test accurately detects the presence of the disease, while the second percentage indicates its accuracy in identifying its absence. According to a 2013 study, during the seasonal rise, these percentages increase to 100% and 95%, respectively [121].

PROCEDURE

- A blood sample is drawn.
- An anticoagulant is added to the blood sample to maintain its liquid state.
- The blood sample is subsequently cooled.
- Through either centrifugation or gravity, the plasma (the liquid component of the blood) is separated from the blood cells.
- Within 48 hours, the chilled sample is dispatched to the laboratory, where the analysis is conducted on the plasma.

REFERENCE VALUES

In 2010, a study was conducted using blood samples from more than 1,000 horses. Based on this, reference values were established that we have been using ever since for horses living in the temperate zone of the northern hemisphere (between the Arctic Circle and the Tropic of Cancer) [26].

This system, which at the time of writing is still the most widely used, assumes two possible outcomes, i.e., PPID likely or unlikely. Between November and July, a horse is deemed PPID-positive if the value surpasses 29 pg/ml (picograms per millilitre); from August-October, the threshold is 47 pg/ml.

There is another system that assumes horses with ACTH levels below 19 pg/ml are unlikely to have PPID, while those above 40 pg/ml are likely to have it. Cases falling between 19 pg/ml and 40 pg/ml are considered equivocal, representing the grey area discussed earlier [160]. It is worth noting that this system is not widely used.

The American College of Veterinary Internal Medicine (ACVIM) has recently established significantly higher cut-off values for diagnosing PPID during the autumn months (see table 1 on the next page).

According to ACVIM, the seasonal rise also starts earlier and runs longer. The peak is still in September and October. This system also differentiates between negative, equivocal, and positive results. The ACVIM-classification is starting to be used increasingly.

The PPID Working Group of the *Equine Endocrinology Group (EEG)* recommends a classification into four periods (table 2).

The *Australian and New Zealand Equine Endocrinology Group (ANZ EEG)* utilises values adjusted for the geographical position in the southern hemisphere when assessing horses in Australia (tables 3 and 4). As of now, there is not enough collected data in New Zealand to conclusively establish reference limits for the diagnosis of PPID.

In all scientific publications on the subject, there's a consistent reminder that blood values should not be straightforwardly extrapolated to match different situations. In the absence of specific values for parts of the southern hemisphere, the current practice is to add about six months to the periods mentioned above.

Don't be overwhelmed by these classifications. Your veterinarian will interpret the blood results based on their chosen classification. If there are any uncertain results, they will pay extra attention to the clinical picture, retest or perform additional tests.

PERIOD	NEGATIVE	EQUIVOCAL	POSITIVE
mid-November – mid-July	< 30 pg/ml	30–50 pg/ml	> 50 pg/ml
mid-July – mid-November	< 50 pg/ml	50–100 pg/ml	> 100 pg/ml

Table 1. ACVIM-values

PERIOD	NEGATIVE	EQUIVOCAL	POSITIVE
December – June	< 15 pg/ml	15–40 pg/ml	> 40 pg/ml
July & November	< 15 pg/ml	15–50 pg/ml	> 50 pg/ml
August	< 20 pg/ml	20–75 pg/ml	> 75 pg/ml
September – October	< 30 pg/ml	30–90 pg/ml	> 90 pg/ml

Table 2. EEG-values

PERIOD	NEGATIVE	EQUIVOCAL	POSITIVE
June – November	< 40 pg/ml	40–70 pg/ml	> 70 pg/ml
December, January, May	< 50 pg/ml	50–80 pg/ml	> 80 pg/ml
February – April	< 80 pg/ml	80–120 pg/ml	> 120 pg/ml

Table 3. ANZ EEG-values – South of and including a latitude of 24° south (southern Queensland)

PERIOD	NEGATIVE	EQUIVOCAL	POSITIVE
June – November	< 55 pg/ml	55–85 pg/ml	> 85 pg/ml
December, January, May	< 80 pg/ml	80–110 pg/ml	> 110 pg/ml
February – April	< 100 pg/ml	100–140 pg/ml	> 140 pg/ml

Table 4. ANZ EEG-values – North of and including a latitude of 20° south (northern Queensland)

Some laboratories use a different value system, counting in pmol/L (picomoles per litre) instead of pg/ml. You can easily convert these values for ACTH yourself:
- To convert from pg/ml to pmol/L, multiply by 0.2202
- To convert from pmol/L to pg/ml, multiply by 4.5413

For example, when discussing blood test results with other horse owners, be sure to specify the value system used to avoid any confusion. Obviously, when comparing repeated test results, it is essential to use the same value.

There are also different analysis techniques (assays) to measure ACTH. You cannot simply compare the results of two blood tests performed by different laboratories, using different techniques [34]. Especially at low ACTH levels, the results of the two techniques diverge.

However, as a horse owner, you need not worry about this complexity. Most commercial labs use the chemiluminescence assay (CIA), while the radioimmunoassay (RIA) is more common in research settings. The ACVIM values, by the way, are based on a CIA. If ever in doubt, you can of course always ask your vet if you can compare the results of the current blood test with those of a previous one.

OTHER FACTORS AFFECTING ACTH

ACTH levels can be influenced by various factors unrelated to PPID. Simply put, your horse might have elevated ACTH without any nerve damage and therefore not have PPID. This is sometimes labelled as pseudo-PPID or pseudo-Cushing's, terms that often contribute more to confusion than to clarity.

For the most reliable results, it is important to have these factors under control as much as possible on the day the blood is drawn. However, this is not always feasible. Factors beyond your control are taken into account by the veterinarian when interpreting the laboratory results.

SEASONAL RISE

From August to October (or mid-July to mid-November with the ACVIM system), higher reference values are employed to determine whether a horse has PPID. This accommodates what is known as the seasonal rise.

The concentration of ACTH in all horses is significantly influenced by day length (or photoperiod). As the days shorten in autumn, there is a notable increase in ACTH production. The cleaving products (alpha-MSH and CLIP) of ACTH, produced by the intermediate lobe, also increase correspondingly. This elevated hormone production is a preparation by the body for the impending food shortage associated with winter.

Whether there is a link in horses between the shortening days and beta-endorphin, directly derived from POMC, has not been firmly established. Building on our knowledge of other mammals and drawing from a 2009 study on mares, it appears logical that the production of this hormone would also increase in the autumn [235]. For convenience, from here on, by seasonal rise we mean the increase in ACTH production in autumn.

In horses with PPID, blood levels during this period are significantly higher compared to healthy horses (see graph). The seasonal rise also tends to persist for a more extended period, particularly in older horses and those with a longer history of the condition.

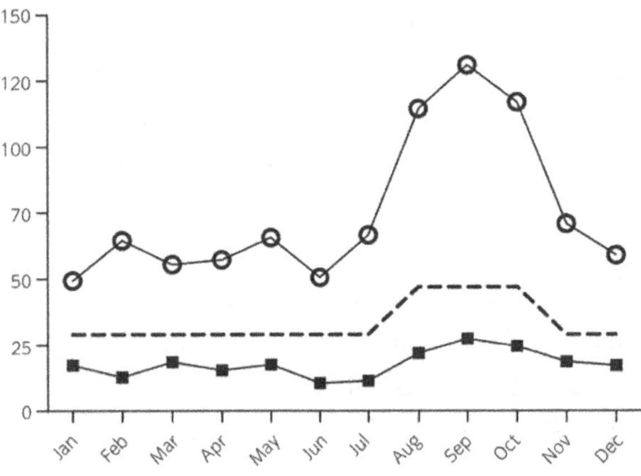

ACTH concentration in pg/ml per month in horses with PPID (circles) and healthy horses (squares). The dotted line indicates the upper limit of the reference values.

(graph: V. Copas, A. Durham [26])

Is testing reliable during this period? Yes, it is indeed quite feasible, as the rise in horses affected by PPID is more pronounced compared to healthy horses. This also facilitates the identification of early cases. When referencing that testing twice a year is recommended, one of these tests should then be conducted during the seasonal rise.

Of course, seasonal rise is not something that happens overnight. It gradually increases at the beginning and then, albeit slightly faster, gradually decreases towards the end. In the periods just before and just after the end of the peak and if the result is inconclusive, it is additionally important to contextualise it within the overall clinical picture. In such cases, a dexamethasone-suppression test (which will be described later) can provide clarity, or you can opt for a retest three months later.

A retrospective study from 2020, utilising a comprehensive database of test results, suggests that reference values should be different even on a weekly basis [29]. Presently, *The Liphook Equine Hospital*, associated with this study, has already implemented this practice. Particularly between June and December, adopting this approach could aid in preventing undetected subclinical cases, ensuring timely treatment. It would also reduce the incidence of horses being treated even though they do not have PPID.

In donkeys and small pony breeds such as Shetland ponies, the seasonal rise is stronger than in horses. In mares, the increase is slightly stronger compared to geldings, and the older the horse, the more pronounced the increase [140].

The number of sunshine hours per day also depends on the latitude at which the horse is located. As we move further north (in the northern hemisphere), the seasonal rise becomes slightly less pronounced [68]. In the southern hemisphere, this is the case as we move further south. The seasonal rise here peaks in March.

Apart from the seasonal rise, hormone levels are pretty much stable. This assumes, of course, that the factors we will discuss shortly are not influencing the situation.

TIME OF DAY

There is a 2014 study that shows that, especially in healthy horses, ACTH is at its highest around eight o'clock in the morning [160]. During the day, it then gradually decreases. Conversely there are also studies showing that this is not the case. The normal, slight fluctuations of ACTH release arise almost exclusively from the anterior lobe of the pituitary gland and therefore distort the picture of ACTH release by the intermediate lobe. This is further underlined by the fact that alpha-MSH, which is derived from the intermediate lobe's ACTH, shows no circadian rhythm.

Nevertheless, to ensure accuracy and facilitate comparison, it is always recommended to conduct repeated tests at around the same time.

> **CIRCADIAN RHYTHM**
> Biological cycle lasting approximately 24 hours, such as the human sleep-wake rhythm.

In healthy horses, ACTH is secreted in pulses by the pituitary gland [178]. This could produce unexpected blood levels. However, the 2014 study did not observe these expected spikes [160]. The researchers suggested that this discrepancy might be attributed to differences in study design.

STRESS

Stress causes higher ACTH levels and thus may confound blood test results [40]. The probability of a false-positive result increases.

In the case of stress, the ACTH stems from the anterior lobe of the pituitary gland; not from the intermediate lobe. With an ACTH test, it is impossible to determine the origin of the measured ACTH.

The act of drawing blood itself can already be so stressful that ACTH goes up. A hurried or grumpy vet, along with a stressed owner, can influence the results. The ride on a trailer to a clinic is also a known stressor. If possible, arrange for blood sampling at home and create a stress-free setting. If your horse needs to be transported on a trailer, wait a minimum of half an hour after unloading before proceeding with blood sampling [93].

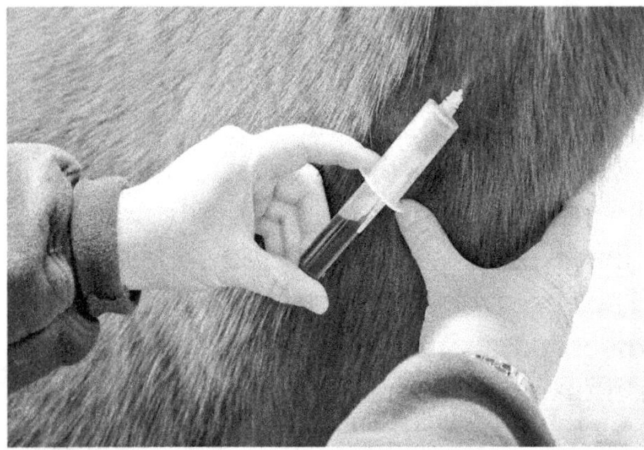

Taking blood can be stressful for your horse

PAIN AND ILLNESS
Pain, akin to stress, triggers an increase in ACTH levels. This ACTH also originates from the anterior lobe of the pituitary gland, providing no information about the presence or absence of PPID. Particularly during the acute phase of laminitis, testing is therefore not recommended. The use of a twitch could also result in higher ACTH levels. So, this is tricky when a horse is twitched for blood sampling.

Horses with PPID are often a bit older, and old age comes with challenges. Age-related ailments, such as osteoarthritis or EOTRH (see page 40), are painful and can thus cause higher ACTH levels.

Seriously ill horses generate substantially higher ACTH levels, rendering ACTH measurement unreliable for diagnosing PPID. Performing this test on a horse with colic, for instance, would void any results; fortunately, no responsible vet would consider doing so.

FOOD
Food intake has a notable impact on ACTH levels. According to a 2014 study, ACTH levels were markedly lower after a 12-hour fasting period, than when measured two hours after food intake, following the same fasting duration [155]. Therefore, ask your vet if they want your horse to have an empty stomach.

A 2018 study found that in healthy, older horses (around 20 years old) being fed a diet high in starch exhibited higher ACTH levels than horses of approximately nine years old on the same diet [65]. This could potentially lead to the misdiagnosis of these healthy seniors as having PPID.

MEDICATION, SEDATION

Horses suffering from respiratory diseases may receive Ventipulmin™ as part of their treatment. This drug is recognised for its potential to elevate ACTH production.

Sedation can cause both increases and decreases in ACTH. According to *The Liphook Equine Hospital,* it is not advisable to sedate a horse to perform an ACTH test [201].

A 2001 Polish study observed lower ACTH levels in rats treated with specific NSAIDs. However, it is unclear whether the same effect occurs in horses [161].

> NSAIDs
>
> Non-steroidal anti-inflammatory drugs. Certain group of analgesic and anti-inflammatory drugs.

EXERCISE

Directly following physical exertion, ACTH production increases [61]. A horse that has just been galloping freely through the pasture or working in the arena will have higher ACTH levels. Take your horse out of the field at least half an hour before the vet's visit and place it in a calm and familiar environment.

HORSE, PONY OR DONKEY, GENDER

In 2010, a study found that donkeys tend to have higher ACTH levels compared to horses, particularly from May to November [250]. A comprehensive 2022 study further supports this finding for Shetland and Welsh ponies (July-September) and Arabians (May-November) [71].

The same study notes that mares exhibit higher ACTH levels in early autumn (September) compared to geldings and stallions. Additional research is required to determine whether and how reference values should be adjusted based on these observed variations.

AGE

As horses age, their ACTH levels tend to increase [140]. This is partly because nerve breakdown is also part of the normal ageing process. One can even question whether an older horse exhibiting age-appropriate nerve breakdown and slightly elevated ACTH levels has PPID, especially if clinical signs remain minimal.

HANDLING OF THE BLOOD SAMPLE

There are a few things your veterinarian should take into account when preparing and sending the blood sample to avoid biased results. Of course, they know very well how to do so and there is no need to point this out to them.

For information some of these factors include: the duration the blood sample is stored before analysis, whether it is properly refrigerated, whether it is frozen or not, the time it is kept frozen and whether TRH-stimulation has been employed or not (we will discuss this further in a moment).

ALPHA-MSH TEST

This is a basal test that measures the amount of alpha-MSH in blood plasma. Alpha-MSH is not affected by things like stress, disease or transport and thus gives fewer false positive or negative results than an ACTH test.

As it is derived from ACTH, alpha-MSH also exhibits a notable increase during the autumn months. This rise is relatively more substantial for alpha-MSH compared to ACTH; up to more than three times higher. Consequently, this test could prove valuable both before and after the peak of the seasonal rise or when the results of an ACTH test are inconclusive. In addition, alpha-MSH may rise early in the disease process, making alpha-MSH testing a more potentially useful tool for early diagnosis.

Measuring alpha-MSH specifically shows that there is a problem in the intermediate lobe, this is not the case with an ACTH test, as ACTH can originate from the frontal lobe as well.

Unfortunately, this test is not yet commercially available. Once it will be, it could become an important diagnostic tool.

BETA-ENDORPHIN TEST

Beta-endorphin is also elevated in PPID. Although it is a cleaving product of POMC, it is not made from ACTH. So, unlike the alpha-MSH determination, a basal beta-endorphin determination says nothing about ACTH.

However, whilst the results of this test could be useful for its reference values, currently there is no laboratory that offers this test commercially. Partly because of this, we still know little about the role of beta-endorphin in relation to PPID.

TRH-STIMULATION TEST

This is a dynamic test that demonstrates an exaggerated response of the pituitary gland to TRH administration in horses with PPID compared to normal horses.

TRH

Thyrotropin-releasing hormone. Hormone produced by the hypothalamus that triggers the pituitary gland's release of certain hormones.

The TRH-stimulation test proves useful when the ACTH results are inconclusive (the equivocal values in the tables on page 76) or when the clinical signs are strongly suggestive of PPID, while the ACTH results are PPID-negative. This test could also be helpful for detecting subclinical PPID. Furthermore, it could be helpful during the period from December to June when ACTH levels are low and exhibit minimal variation. Lastly, it could play a decisive role in aforementioned cases where ACTH elevation is caused by factors other than PPID.

Like ACTH determination, the TRH-stimulation test is subject to fluctuating values that depend on season, age, stress, and food intake.

Research published in 2020 suggests that this test can be performed in horses with mild to moderate pain without affecting the outcome [19].

The test could serve as an adjunct to the dexamethasone-suppression test (DST) described below if the latter has been performed previously and proving inconclusive. The TRH-stimulation test is therefore well suited to demonstrate PPID at an early stage.

PROCEDURE
- Blood is drawn as described for the ACTH-test to measure ACTH and optionally alpha-MSH.
- Then 1 mg of TRH is administered intravenously (0.5 mg for ponies lighter than 250 kg / 550 lbs).
- After 10 minutes, a second blood sample is taken.
- In horses with PPID, ACTH is now substantially higher; alpha-MSH is even four times higher.
- In some circumstances, after 30 minutes, a third sample is taken and analysed.

Seasonal variations in response to TRH are observed in healthy horses. Consequently, it is advisable not to conduct this test from August to October. Furthermore, proper reference values for this period have not been established yet.

DEXAMETHASONE-SUPPRESSION TEST (DST)

Dexamethasone is a synthetic variant of cortisol. Cortisol has an inhibitory effect on the anterior lobe of the pituitary gland. Administering dexamethasone artificially inhibits it from producing ACTH. The adrenal glands will now produce less cortisol. The extent to which cortisol production decreases can be measured in the blood.

If it is insufficient after administration of dexamethasone, this is an indication that the intermediate lobe of the pituitary gland is producing a lot of ACTH. In a healthy horse, this will not be the case; in a horse with PPID, it will. Simply put, with this dynamic test you temporarily switch off the major source of cortisol, allowing you to see what the other, smaller source is doing.

Given that the body's endogenous cortisol production persists and is subject to various uncontrollable factors, the DST may yield both false-positive and false-negative results. This test was once considered the gold standard, but that is no longer the case today.

The test necessitates the administration of synthetic corticosteroids, which is inadvisable for horses with PPID teetering on the brink of laminitis or already affected by it. Particularly in these cases, it would be beneficial to use the TRH-stimulation test.

A practical inconvenience is that the veterinarian has to visit twice.

PROCEDURE
- Blood is drawn around four in the afternoon to determine cortisol levels.
- A small amount (40 µg/kg body weight) of dexamethasone is then injected into a vein.
- The following day, blood is drawn again around noon. For a negative test result, the cortisol level in this blood sample must be low.

There are no proper reference values established that state how much lower the cortisol levels must be.

The 2018 study mentioned on page 80 not only saw higher ACTH levels in old horses on a high-starch diet, but also noted elevated cortisol levels [65]. This should be taken into account when employing the dexamethasone-suppression test.

For the diagnosis of PPID in donkeys, this test does not seem suitable, as it yields too many false-negative results [123].

DOMPERIDONE-RESPONSE TEST
Domperidone is a dopamine antagonist. That is, it has an inhibitory effect on dopamine. Following administration, the intermediate lobe of the pituitary gland of PPID-affected horses will produce much more ACTH [38]. In healthy horses, this will not be the case because for them the anterior lobe of the pituitary gland is the main source of ACTH. The anterior lobe is not under the influence of dopamine. This dynamic test is less commonly employed nowadays.

TESTING FOR INSULIN DYSREGULATION

Insulin dysregulation affects at least one in three horses with PPID. Consequently, it is important to at least once test for insulin and glucose levels in the blood, or have an oral glucose tolerance test done. Timely diagnosis and management of insulin dysregulation plays a key role in reducing the risk of laminitis and exacerbation of EMS.

A horse in pain, for example due to laminitis, or a horse in stress, produces more cortisol and adrenaline [40]. This has an impact on the concentrations of glucose, insulin, and leptin in the blood. It is therefore advisable to postpone testing until the pain and stress are significantly lower. However, this can be challenging, especially considering that mandatory fasting for the fasting insulin determination, as described below, may also induce stress.

> **ADRENALINE**
> Hormone and neurotransmitter that affects blood sugar levels, among other things.

If blood results for insulin dysregulation worsen unexpectedly in repeated tests, it could signal that a horse, initially diagnosed with insulin dysregulation, might now also be developing PPID.

INSULIN TEST

This is a basal test, of which there are two variants. In one, the horse must be fasted; in the other, this is not necessary.

FASTING INSULIN TEST

In fasting insulin testing, blood is drawn after a six-hour fasting period. The concentration of insulin in the blood sample is subsequently assessed. Insulin levels exceeding 20 IU/L are categorised as hyperinsulinaemic for the majority of breeds [52].

> **IU/L**
> International units per litre. Pharmaceutical unit of measurement for a relative quantity of a substance.

The insulin response (peak insulin production) is affected by numerous factors. This test therefore yields many false negatives [223]. In other words, the wrong conclusion is drawn that there is no insulin resistance. This is because this is a snapshot test taken during a fasting period where food intake which would normally trigger the body's insulin response has been eliminated. Thus, the test does not reveal how your horse would respond to sugar ingestion. Nearly two out of three insulin-resistant horses slip through this test. The number of false-positive results is also high.

The upper cut-off value in the fasting insulin test can be different for some horse breeds. Your veterinarian will take this into account.

NON-FASTING INSULIN TEST

In the non-fasting insulin test, the horse is not required to fast in the six hours preceding blood extraction and has access to grass or hay. Similar to the previous test, the amount of insulin in the blood sample is measured. The major drawback is that the precise amount of carbohydrates consumed is unknown. If there was a lot of sugar in the food, the insulin response will also be high.

This test is less accurate than the fasting insulin test. To address this, attempts have been made to enhance accuracy by increasing the upper limit of the reference values by half. It is deemed impossible for a non-insulin-resistant horse to exceed this adjusted limit through normal eating. However, there are many equivocal cases just below the upper limit. An advantage of the non-fasting insulin test is that it produces fewer false-negative results.

INSULIN-RESPONSE TEST

Of this dynamic test, there are also two versions; the two-step insulin-response test and the combined glucose-insulin test.

TWO-STEP INSULIN-RESPONSE TEST

In the two-step insulin-response test, the initial step involves measuring the baseline glucose level in the blood. Subsequently, the veterinarian administers insulin to the horse. After half an hour, the blood glucose is measured once more. In horses without insulin dysregulation, the glucose level should be at least halved. Conversely, in horses with insulin dysregulation, this is not the case.

COMBINED GLUCOSE-INSULIN TEST (CGIT)

The combined glucose-insulin test is a variant of the two-step insulin response test, wherein glucose is injected, followed by insulin. After three-quarters of an hour, blood sugar levels are measured. These should then be back to normal in horses without insulin dysregulation. Another half-hour later, a similar assessment is done for insulin levels, which should also have returned to normal.

Both the two-step insulin-response test and the combined glucose-insulin test, are mainly used in a scientific context and within specialised equine clinics.

LEPTIN AND ADIPONECTIN TEST

The veterinarian can also measure the amount of the appetite-regulating hormone leptin in the blood. On page 41 we have covered insulin resistance; in the early stages of insulin resistance, blood sugar levels remain fairly normal, while the amount of insulin in the blood is too high. Nevertheless, insulin levels may remain just within the reference values. An elevated leptin level would then be the deciding factor; proving that there is insulin dysregulation.

The levels of adiponectin can also be determined. Horses with insulin dysregulation are more likely to have reduced adiponectin levels.

High leptin levels along with low adiponectin levels are predictive of the occurrence of laminitis in ponies, according to a 2017 study [219].

Your veterinarian would normally only administer these tests if previous test results were still inconclusive.

SERUM GLUCOSE TEST

This is a basal test that assesses the sugar levels in the blood serum. It is considered more accurate than measuring sugar levels directly in the blood.

> **BLOOD SERUM**
> Bright yellow liquid obtained by allowing blood plasma to clot and then subjecting the clot to centrifugation.

ORAL GLUCOSE-TOLERANCE TEST (OGTT)

The unreliability of basal fasting insulin test can be overcome with the dynamic oral glucose-tolerance test (or oral sugar test/OST) as it yields fewer false negatives [33].

The test aims to illustrate how sugar is processed in the body and whether hormonal problems occur in the process. Two blood samples are collected. One after a six-hour fasting period and the other following the administration of a measured dose of sugar syrup. This amount of sugar is much higher than that which could be ingested through normal grazing. If insulin levels shoot up after glucose administration, then insulin resistance is most likely present.

OTHER TESTS

For completeness, we mention the cortisol determination and the ACTH-stimulation test. These two tests are used less and less. In fact, the *PPID Working Group* of *The Equine Endocrinology Group* (EEG) even states that they are unsuitable for the diagnosis of PPID [222].

CORTISOL TEST

Measuring the amount of cortisol in blood, saliva or urine is not conclusive, as equines affected by PPID typically do not exhibit elevated cortisol levels.

In light of recent studies it would be preferable to measure free cortisol. These days, science is also looking at other abnormalities in cortisol metabolism (see 'Cortisol dysregulation' on page 24). Moreover, there are all sorts of other conditions and circumstances that can affect cortisol levels such as stress, pain, other diseases, strenuous exercise, medication, sedation, time of year and time of day.

An advantage of a urine or saliva test is that they do not induce stress, as can a blood test. The act of drawing blood can intrinsically elevate cortisol levels due to stress, potentially distorting the test results.

Previously, deviations in the normal variations within blood cortisol levels throughout the day were also looked at; the so-called circadian rhythm. It was believed that elevated ACTH levels might disrupt this rhythm. There is a possibility that ACTH produced from the intermediate lobe is biologically less active (although opinions vary, see page 25) and therefore has little influence on cortisol production. Moreover, the circadian rhythm typically diminishes with illness and is a component of the natural aging process.

ACTH-STIMULATION TEST

This is a dynamic test in which ACTH is administered. This triggers increased cortisol production by the adrenal glands. The larger the adrenal glands, the greater the cortisol production. Thus, in horses with enlarged adrenal glands, more cortisol is released after ACTH stimulation than in healthy horses. Adrenal enlargement is rare in PPID-afflicted equines. Therefore, this test is only limited usefulness unless it is employed specifically to determine adrenal enlargement.

MEDICAL IMAGING

Medical imaging in the context of scientific research has provided us with considerable knowledge and insight. In practice, it is less common unless applied to visualise certain clinical signs.

RADIOGRAPHY

Radiographs (X-rays) are useful in the context of laminitis (see sidebar 'Recognising laminitis' on page 69). They are particularly valuable for evaluating the reduction of coffin bone rotation, a positive sign of your horse's recovery.

Larger hoof abscesses are visible on x-rays as well. Osteoporosis can also be shown from a certain degree of degeneration onwards.

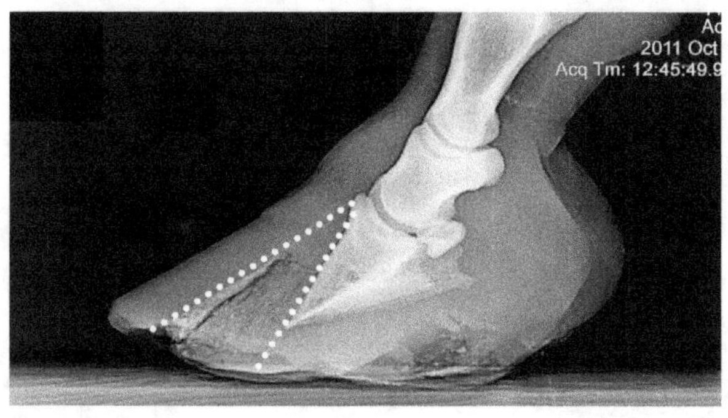

Radiograph showing a coffin bone rotation
(*photo: Myhre Equine Clinic*)

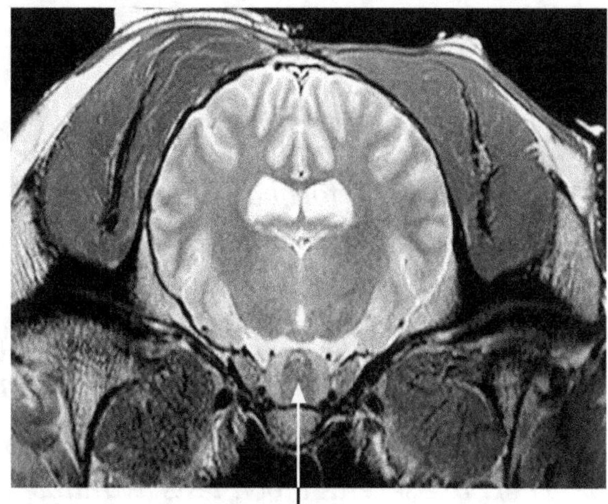

MRI showing an enlarged pituitary gland
(*photo: University of Veterinary Medicine Hanover*)

MRI

Magnetic Resonance Imaging (MRI) is a technique that employs magnetic waves to visualise organs, joints, and more. It can be used to detect pituitary gland enlargement, as well as compression of surrounding brain tissue.

However, an MRI does not provide information on whether and to what extent the abnormalities found will have a negative impact. There are horses with pituitary enlargement without clinical signs and vice versa.

Getting an MRI scan is costly and the horse needs to be anaesthetised. It is highly uncommon for a vet to opt for this diagnostic tool. Evaluating the clinical signs in combination with one or more blood tests will actually prove to be conclusive in the vast majority of cases.

POST-MORTEM EXAMINATION

Post-mortem examination (autopsy) can reveal adenomas, pituitary enlargement, and damage to surrounding brain structures due to pressure from the distended pituitary gland. In older horses, adenomas may be found even when there were no clinical manifestations of PPID during their lifetime. Adrenal enlargement is also a potential finding.

Post-mortem examination is done almost exclusively to gain scientific knowledge about PPID.

SUMMARY

To make the correct diagnosis of PPID, the veterinarian will conduct an anamnesis, perform a clinical examination and do blood tests. The latter to test for both PPID and EMS/insulin dysregulation.

The anamnesis is a comprehensive questioning interview primarily centred on clinical signs. The clinical examination proceeds from this initial assessment, with special emphasis on scrutinising laminitis associated with PPID, as it can be inconspicuous in the early stages.

There are several blood tests available to diagnose PPID, with the ACTH test being the most frequently utilised. This entails measuring the amount of ACTH in the blood. Autumn is the best time to do this, as this is when the rise in ACTH is greatest in horses affected by PPID.

ACTH production can also be triggered by other factors. These should be eliminated as much as possible for a more reliable test result. When in doubt, the veterinarian can use other tests, although not all of these are yet widely adopted.

Various blood tests are available, with a particular focus on assessing insulin dysregulation, to diagnose Equine Metabolic Syndrome (EMS).

Medical imaging and post-mortem examinations are predominantly conducted for scientific purposes.

TREATMENT

PPID is a complicated condition that impacts the entire system of a horse. Treating it involves addressing the horse as a whole. Unfortunately, surgically removing a pituitary adenoma in horses isn't feasible. These days, medication is the accepted norm for treatment. A good veterinarian will thoroughly inform clients about this medication and other treatment choices.

In reality, treatment also involves paying more attention to overall health care and making adjustments to living conditions to enhance the well-being of older horses. Your role as an owner in this process is crucial. Once treatment begins, the vet should closely monitor its effectiveness.

EMS/INSULIN DYSREGULATION

You know now that PPID and EMS/ID can coexist in a horse, and they are not entirely unrelated. However, the scientific community recommends diagnosing and treating both conditions separately as distinct illnesses.

COMPLICATIONS

Of course, complications clearly defined by clinical signs must also be treated. This requires focus on proper nutrition, regular hoof, coat and dental care, worming, vaccination, and ensuring sufficient exercise. All of which requires a great deal of organisation.

Getting together a good team of practitioners (vet, hoof care provider, dentist, nutritionist), who broadly share the same vision is vital. Consistent advice is essential for your horse to receive optimal care.

Keep a close eye on your horse's weight (see sidebar 'Determining body weight' on page 93) and record it in the log mentioned on page 27.

When assessing improvements in the clinical picture, the response to treatment often appears first and most prominently as a reduction in hypertrichosis and the severity of laminitis.

Other positive changes may include a decrease or disappearance of hyper/hypohidrosis, infections, inflammation, apathy, exercise intolerance, muscle atrophy, the pendulous belly, polyuria, polydipsia, and the onset of intended weight loss.

Again: PPID is a complicated syndrome. Don't expect yourself to suddenly become a PPID expert after diagnosis and initiation of treatment. Therefore, explicitly ask your vet for guidance on the pathway to follow now.

MEDICATIONS

PPID cannot be cured. Medication, however, can slow down and sometimes halt the disease. Furthermore, there are drugs that can help reduce the consequential damage (secondary disorders or complications) of PPID. Let's begin by examining the first group of medications.

DOPAMINE AGONISTS

A dopamine agonist is a substance that resembles dopamine in its action. It activates dopamine receptors in the pituitary gland. Giving dopamine agonists will inhibit the production of POMC and thus the release of melanocortins by the intermediate lobe.

Simply put, a dopamine agonist replaces the missing body's own dopamine. This causes the horse's pituitary gland to hit the brakes and decrease hormone production. Since PPID is irreversible, a dopamine agonist will have to be given for life.

Apart from the fact that dopamine agonists can reduce certain clinical signs, they can also delay further nerve degradation [191]. Waiting too long to start this medication is therefore not recommended.

There is no evidence yet that dopamine agonists can completely stop nerve degradation. Reversing the damage is all but out of the question.

It is not yet known whether this drug also slows pituitary enlargement in PPID horses. Because this is theoretically quite likely, but more so because this phenomenon is so undesirable, we should take this into account when considering starting medication. However, we should point out that a 2020 study found no difference in the size of the pituitary gland between PPID-affected horses who received treatment and those who did not [228]. On the other hand, the study population was small and the comparisons were made after only six months of medication.

In humans, treatment with dopamine agonists has been shown to decrease the size of adenomas in the anterior lobe of the pituitary gland (prolactinomas) [49]. This, of course, does not mean that this kite also holds true for adenomas in the intermediate lobe of the pituitary gland of horses.

DETERMINING BODY WEIGHT

Embracing the formula that knowledge is derived from measurement understanding the weight of your horse is beneficial. While a weighbridge will provide the exact weight, you can also use this method:

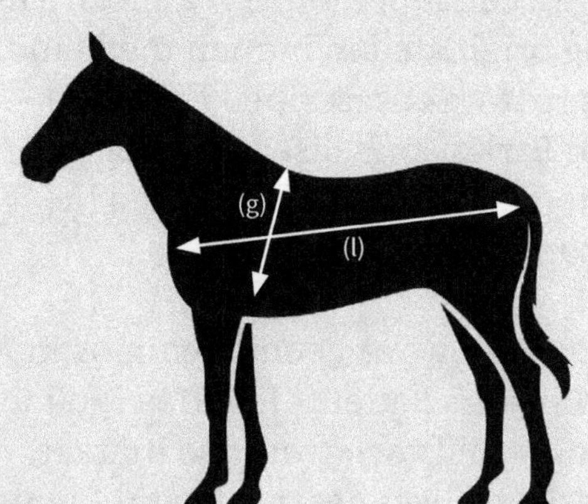

- Measure the girth (g) of your horse's chest just behind his forelegs.
- Measure the body length (l) from the sternum (point of the chest) to the ischium (point of the buttock).
- The horse's weight is calculated by a formula that uses a constant which depends on the system you use, metric or imperial.
- The formula has a margin of 10%.
- **Metric system**
  (girth squared x body length), divided by 11,900
  Example: Girth 170 cm, length 210 cm
  ((170 x 170) x 210) / 11,900
  This horse weighs 510 kilos.
- **Imperial system**
  (girth squared x body length), divided by 330
  Example: Girth 67", length 83"
  ((67 x 67) x 83) / 330
  This horse weighs 1129 lbs.

Determining the weight by using a weight tape is the least accurate method. You might be 65 kilos (143 lbs) wrong with this method. So that could be either 65 kilos too much or too little.

Now you have to compare this with what is a normal weight for the breed. These are roughly the weight margins for the most common breeds in kilos, (lbs in brackets):

- Miniature horse: 100 - 200 (220 - 440)
- Shetland pony: 150 - 250 (330 - 550)
- Welsh, Exmoor, New Forest pony: 250 - 400 (220 - 440)
- Icelandic: 300 - 450 (660 - 990)
- Arabian: 400 - 500 (880 - 1100)
- Fjord, Haflinger: 450 - 600 (990 - 1320)
- Warmblood: 500 - 700 (1100 - 1540)
- Frisian, Irish cob: 500 - 800 (1100 - 1760)
- Draught horse: 700 and heavier (1540 and up)

PERGOLIDE

The dopamine agonist of choice in PPID is pergolide mesylate. From here on, we call it pergolide for short. The drug originated in human medicine, where it was prescribed to people with Parkinson's disease; a nervous system disorder characterised by dopamine deficiency.

In 2007, however, complications in Parkinson's patients led to pergolide being withdrawn from the market. These involved heart valve problems. It's important to note that such complications have not been observed in horses.

BLOOD VALUES

After the initial dose, both ACTH, alpha-MSH, CLIP, and beta-endorphin decrease within 48 hours [16]. Following two months of treatment, about 30% of horses exhibit ACTH levels within the reference values. Nearly 60% experience a decrease, although their levels remain above the upper limit. Pergolide thus lowers ACTH concentrations in most cases [95].

In just over 10% of horses, there is no observed change after two months. For these cases, a gradual increase in dosage is often considered. Patience is also important. Some horses with PPID respond to the medication only after a longer period of time.

CLINICAL PICTURE

Approximately 75% of horses treated with pergolide demonstrate clinical improvement within four to eight weeks. Specifically, issues like coat problems, sweating, polydipsia/polyuria, and the pot belly tend to diminish. Unfortunately, according to a 2021 study, it does not look like it may not enhance immune function in horses with PPID [89].

Despite a 2021 study suggesting that pergolide hasn't been conclusively proven to impact muscle mass loss (atrophy) [169], many veterinarians and horse owners report improvements in this area. It's worth noting that the failure to observe a reduction in muscle atrophy with pergolide in the study might be attributed to the relatively short test period (12 weeks).

Pergolide reduces hypertriglyceridaemia (elevated blood fat levels) associated with EMS. Body weight also improves [169]. Insulin levels do not improve according to most studies [89, 94, 247].

Mares with PPID suffering from irregular oestrus (heat) or infertility may also benefit from this drug [103, 247].

Research from 2018 states that there is still insufficient evidence to definitively conclude that treatment with pergolide reduces the risk of the occurrence or recurrence of laminitis in horses with PPID [57].

Other studies do report an improvement in the clinical signs of laminitis when treated with pergolide. However, these improvements cannot be attributed one-to-one to pergolide. Other factors such as hoof care and adjustments in nutrition, housing and exercise also play a major role.

Available brands

Pergolide is commercialised under the brand name Prascend®. It was the only dopamine agonist allowed to be prescribed for veterinary use in 2012. The use of Permax®, Celance®, and other drugs prescribed in human medicine for Parkinson's disease has not been allowed since then.

In 2019, the drug Pergoquin™ entered the UK and EU market. Its mechanism of action is identical to that of Prascend®. In 2021, the drug Pergocoat™/Pergosafe™ was added as a third option.

In the UK, pergolide is also available in an unlicensed paste form, manufactured by Bova. In the US, the only FDA-approved pergolide formulation for horses is still Prascend®. Compounded pergolide formulations are also available, but their effectiveness and stability have been shown to vary.

Dosage

The recommended dose is 0.002 mg (2 μg)/kilo body weight once daily. So, for a 500-kilo (1100 lbs) horse, that is one milligram tablet.

Because pergolide has a short half-life, so dividing the dose in half and giving it twice daily, would be even better [194]. This approach minimises fluctuations of the drug in the blood. As far as possible, always administer pergolide at the same time each day. This also prevents fluctuations.

> ### Half-life
> The time required for a quantity of a substance in the body to reduce to half of its initial value. It is an indicator of the duration of action.

As the horse get older, the dosage may often need to be increased. The same goes for cases where the disease progresses into an advanced stage. Some horses may require up to 5 mg per day [99].

Some veterinarians base the dosage not solely on standard guidelines but on the horse's individual condition. They argue that the right dosage is the one that brings ACTH levels back to normal, even if it exceeds the manufacturer's recommended maximum dose.

In many cases, the dosage can be adjusted downwards after the drug takes effect. This is even recommended to minimise side effects. Take this decision in consultation with your vet, after it has been established that the clinical signs have diminished and blood tests have shown that the drug also appears to be effective on a hormonal level in your horse.

Because of the half-life, you do have to keep giving it every day. So, if you are going to halve starting from 1 mg, give half a tablet every day and not a whole tablet every other day. Otherwise, there will be fluctuations in blood levels. What is also commonly done is to start on a low dose and then slowly build up. Again: make sure to consult with your veterinarian.

The pills feature a break line, allowing you to easily administer half doses. For smaller amounts, consider using a pill splitter. Pergoquin™ tablets have two break lines, making it simpler to divide them into quarters.

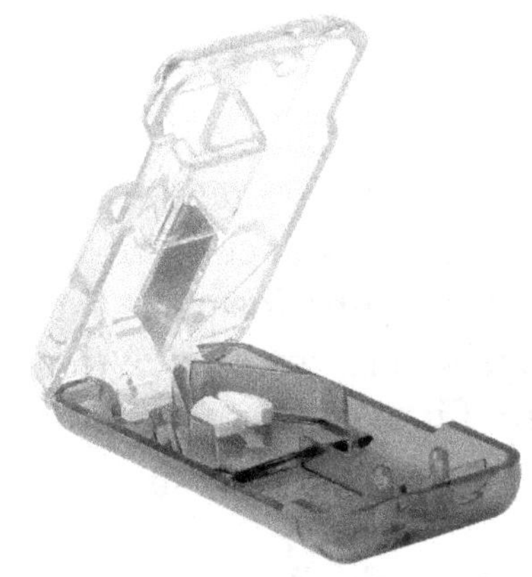

Pill splitter

Pergocoat™/Pergosafe™ is a film-coated tablet that can not be split. It exists in 0.5 / 1 / 2 mg doses.

In England, as mentioned, pergolide is on the market in paste form. This form of administration has advantages that can make a significant difference for some horses. Even so significant that this might count as a clinical justification for preferring an unlicensed drug to a licensed one. Some horses absolutely resist tablet administration. Using this paste might be more effective, given its more pleasant taste compared to pills. Moreover, the syringe is calibrated in 0.2 mg increments, helping to prevent or manage side effects effectively. Administering half the dose twice a day is an option as well. For small, light ponies, precise dosing would be highly beneficial.

Unlicensed means that the medication has not been given a license for this specific use in horses, but it can still be prescribed by a vet under certain circumstances. It is important to note that the licensing status of a medication doesn't necessarily reflect its safety or effectiveness.

During the seasonal rise, you could increase the dosage [193]. This approach may prevent the recurrence of previously resolved clinical signs. In mid-November, you can revert the horse to its regular dosage. Certain horses suffer so little from their PPID that they may only need medication during the seasonal rise.

The pills can be kept for two years without losing their efficacy. Should you buy over from another horse owner, verify the expiry date.

ADJUSTMENTS IN MEDICATION

After a month on the medication, have blood tests and clinical examinations conducted again to assess whether adjustments, either up or down, are necessary. Increasing the dose is done in increments of 0.5 mg every two to four weeks.

The table below shows how to react to the different combinations of blood values and changes in clinical picture.

Some horse owners reason that the clinical picture is more important than the blood values. What they overlook in doing so is that it is mainly the easily observable clinical signs that they see improving, such as better shedding or less drinking, urination and sweating. Unfortunately, the increased risk of laminitis and infections remains invisible until it is too late.

	STABILISATION OR IMPROVEMENT OF THE CLINICAL PICTURE	NO STABILISATION OR IMPROVEMENT OF THE CLINICAL PICTURE
IMPROVED BLOOD TEST RESULTS	Another blood test and clinical examination every three to six months to see if dosage can be lowered. At least one of those examinations in autumn, during the seasonal rise.	Especially if secondary problems arise, such as laminitis, infections or weight loss, they should be looked at first to see if they can be solved differently rather than increasing the dosage.
NO IMPROVED BLOOD TEST RESULTS	Some vets will want to increase the dosage to prevent pituitary enlargement. Others will keep the dosage unchanged to avoid side effects.	The dose is increased and eventually complemented with cyproheptadine (see page 101). Wait at least two months after starting the medication before making this adjustment.

HOW TO ADMINISTER

It is literally a bitter pill for some horses. There are a few tricks you can try to get it to take its medication anyway:

- Little bit of mash in the middle of a feeder with the pill pressed in. Make sure your horse actually eats it and does not leave it in the trough. You don't want another horse to accidentally ingest the medicine.
- Make a slit in a piece of carrot and put the pill in there.
- Put the pill in the back of the cheek or on the back of the tongue.
- Dissolve it in water and then squirt it into the back of the mouth with a syringe. This is done as follows:
  - Remove the plunger and put the medicine in the syringe. You can grind the pill with a clean mortar first.
  - Block the end of the syringe with your finger.
  - Add water (about 50 ml) and put the plunger back in the syringe. Shake well until the medicine is completely dissolved in the water.
  - Halter your horse. Hold the syringe at the side between the horse's lips and squirt the contents on the back of its tongue.
  - Hold its head up until it has swallowed the water.
  - If it won't swallow, rub your thumb against the side of its tongue. Most horses then get a swallowing reflex.

Use disposable gloves when handling the pill, or wash your hands after administration. Especially if you break or pulverise the pills (which you should not do according to the instructions, by the way), to prevent potential eye irritation or headaches.

HOW QUICKLY IT WORKS

If the medicine takes effect well, we see improvement in the first four to eight weeks. The horse becomes livelier and shows less apathy. The will to work bounces back. Issues with sweating decrease, as do polyuria and polydipsia. ACTH levels decrease, although they may remain too high. Glucose and insulin measurements sometimes also give better results, even though most studies say that no effect on insulin levels is to be expected.

In a 2002 field study, 85% of horse owners reported an improvement in clinical signs after treatment with pergolide [247].

Over the next few months, we see improvement with regard to coat problems. To draw any firm conclusions about shedding improvement, you will have to wait for spring.

Muscling in the back improves. The pendulous belly will be less prominent, despite the results of previous research to the contrary [169]. The horse suffers less from recurrent inflammations and abscesses. Laminitis either lessens in severity or happens less often, despite the 2018 study indicating a lack of compelling scientific evidence supporting this claim [120].

Should your horse be left without pergolide once due to circumstances, ACTH levels will begin to rise again after about 48 hours. Deterioration of clinical signs occurs much less quickly [222].

SIDE EFFECTS

Although a 2012 study says that horse owners' satisfaction with pergolide is mostly good and another 2019 study concludes that the drug is generally well tolerated, there are certain known side effects that we should not underestimate [51, 193]. There is much debate among horse owners about the extent to which side effects should factor into the decision to give pergolide, but there's no clear-cut answer to this dilemma. The reality is the disease is both progressive and irreversible. Therefore, without administering the drug, the condition will almost certainly worsen. Yet, in certain horses, the side effects can be so severe that this situation is also deemed unacceptable. Sometimes, the decision needs to be made by balancing the horse's quality of life against its life expectancy.

Pregnant mares can receive pergolide treatment, although there is a risk of prolonged gestation or a detached placenta [80]. One month before foaling, the dosage should be tapered off to avoid lack of milk yield. If the milk production is satisfactory in both quantity and quality, the medication can be reintroduced one month after foaling.

Not enough research data exist yet to say anything meaningful about possible long-term side effects. However, studies tracking horses for over five years have not reported such effects [131, 168].

PERGOLIDE VEIL

Despite the aforementioned dosing preferences, accurately dosing pergolide poses a challenge. Overdosing may occur, leading to a synthetic dopamine surplus. Approximately one in three horses loose appetite (anorexia) or show signs of apathy upon starting or increasing the recommended dose, as indicated by a study [95]. This is commonly referred to as the 'pergolide veil'.

It is best to pause the medication for two to three days. Then begin anew with half of the dose. Gradually increase the dosage thereafter. Always consult your vet before making these adjustments.

The reduced appetite is usually transient and tends to vanish within six weeks. It is also fortunately not constant in most horses. In other words, horses often show moments during the day when they are willing to eat. Apathy remains a problem in some horses even when appetite returns. This is often mentioned as a reason why people decide to stop giving the medication.

Behavioural change

Aggression is not mentioned as a side effect in the package leaflet. Nevertheless, this behavioural change is observed by some horse owners. The supposed explanation for this is that pergolide, as intended, causes a decrease in POMC and hence beta-endorphin. Since beta-endorphin is a powerful endogenous opiate-like substance that is analgesic and anti-inflammatory, a reduction in its levels might intensify the perception of pain related to PPID complications. Consequently, the horse might exhibit aggressive behaviour in response.

Restlessness, nervous behaviour and increased activity also occur and may also be linked to altered hormone levels.

Diarrhea

Diarrhea occurs in about 30% of horses and can be dealt with in the same way as the pergolide veil [95]. Hold off medication for a few days and then slowly build up from a lower dose.

Colic

Some horses show mild colic symptoms, typically resolving without intervention.

Interaction with other substances

Acepromazine is a drug that has vasodilatory and blood pressure-lowering effects. It is sometimes prescribed for laminitis. Horses with PPID treated with pergolide should not also be given acepromazine. Pergolide is a dopamine agonist; acepromazine is a dopamine antagonist. These medications have opposing effects and counteract each other's actions.

Mares that have just foaled are sometimes given domperidone to stimulate milk production, if not naturally. This drug is a dopamine antagonist and therefore inhibits dopamine. As a result, it increases ACTH production in the intermediate lobe of the pituitary gland. According to the package leaflet of Prascend™, domperidone may reduce the action of pergolide.

Cabergoline

This is a dopamine agonist that is available in a slow-release intramuscular injectable form. Each dose is a small 1 ml injection and lasts for about 14 days. This form of administration can be particularly useful for horses that are difficult to medicate orally.

However, not all horses respond adequately to the 1 ml dose, and adjustments may be necessary. In the UK injectable cabergoline is unlicensed; in the US it is licensed.

As with any medication, cabergoline can have potential side effects. They are similar to those of pergolide, but they are not predictable from the horse's response to pergolide. There may be more or fewer side effects when switching between drugs. Side effects usually last for 1 to 3 days following an injection. One common side effect of cabergoline is a temporary loss of appetite. This effect is usually short-lived, with the horse's normal appetite returning within 7-10 days. However, if their appetite doesn't bounce back once their body gets used to the drug, it's advisable to consult with a vet. They may need to adjust the dose.

BROMOCRIPTINE

Bromocriptine, a dopamine agonist sold under the brand name Parlodel™, is not recommended due to its side effects. Anorexia is one of the mentioned side effects. Moreover, it has inferior oral absorption compared to pergolide. Additionally, its half-life is shorter than that of pergolide.

Recent research has found that the drug can lower insulin sensitivity. Not a helpful feature given that a large proportion of horses with PPID suffer from insulin dysregulation [76].

SEROTONIN ANTAGONISTS

A serotonin antagonist is a substance that limits the activity of serotonin receptors, thereby making the body less responsive to serotonin. Studies in rats indicate that serotonin stimulates the release of ACTH in the intermediate lobe of the pituitary gland. The drug cyproheptadine has been demonstrated to suppress this response [46].

> **SEROTONIN**
> Hormone and neurotransmitter that affects the sleep cycle, sexual activity and appetite, among other things. It also plays a role in processing pain stimuli.

CYPROHEPTADINE

The drug cyproheptadine is one such serotonin antagonist. It was one of the first drugs employed in combating PPID. If the maximum dose of pergolide turns out to be insufficient in suppressing clinical signs, veterinarians may prescribe cyproheptadine. It is marketed under the brand name Periactin™.

There are studies showing that in terms of improvement of clinical signs, no more effect can be expected from cyproheptadine than from changes in living conditions.

It is sometimes claimed that cyproheptadine and pergolide are mutually reinforcing. No substantial research has validated this assertion.

In the 2002 field study mentioned, 85% of owners of horses treated with pergolide reported clinical improvement, contrasting with only 28% of those using cyproheptadine [247].

SIDE EFFECTS

Horses can become drowsy and sleepy from cyproheptadine. In mice, cyproheptadine use has been shown to make them more susceptible to epileptic seizures [216]. In horses with PPID affected by this neurological problem, the drug is therefore less frequently prescribed. Finally, ataxia (muscle dysfunction) occurs in some horses treated with cyproheptadine. As this is also a possible complication in horses with advanced PPID, the same applies here: caution is advised.

ENZYME INHIBITING DRUGS

TRILOSTANE

Adrenal enlargement (adrenal hyperplasia and hypertrophy) may occur in horses with advanced PPID. This increases cortisol production (hypercortisolaemia). To inhibit this process, the drug trilostane may be prescribed. It works by inhibiting the enzyme responsible for converting cholesterol into cortisol.

In particular, polyuria and polydipsia are clinical signs that diminish with use. Good results are also seen with regard to laminitis. Apathy also decreases [96].

It's important to note that trilostane may weaken the horse's natural defenses. Considering that horses with PPID commonly experience immune system disturbances, veterinarians exercise caution when prescribing trilostane.

SELEGILINE

In certain cases, dopamine agonists are combined with synthetic enzyme inhibitors to slow down the breakdown of dopamine, extending its impact. Occasionally, they're employed to postpone the use of pergolide for a while. Although these drugs alleviate clinical signs to some extent, they do not solve the problem. Selegiline is one such drug.

DRUGS FOR SECONDARY CONDITIONS

As discussed thoroughly in the 'Description' chapter, horses affected by PPID often experience various secondary conditions or complications. Let's now explore some medications that can be utilised to treat these conditions.

ANTIBIOTIC DRUGS

The secondary infections mentioned on page 35, often require treatment with antibiotic drugs. Early and vigorous intervention is the message. Even minor infections can quickly become difficult to control in PPID-affected horses.

Antibiotics are often prescribed in laminitis to reduce inflammation of the dermal lamellae (page 49). Only, this is a sterile inflammation. In simpler terms, it's inflammation without the presence of bacteria. So, the use of antibiotics is somewhat futile. However, in cases of sole perforation accompanied by inflammation, antibiotic treatment becomes necessary.

ANALGESIC AND ANTI-INFLAMMATORY DRUGS

Most pain-relieving medications also have anti-inflammatory properties. They are NSAIDs (Non-Steroidal Anti-Inflammatory Drugs). Commonly prescribed drugs include phenylbutazone ('bute' or Equipalazone™), flunixin (Banamine™), and ketoprofen (Dinalgen™). These are so-called non-selective NSAIDs.

Possible complications from excessive use of these types of NSAIDs are stomach ulcers, intestinal inflammation, liver and kidney problems, fluid retention, and blood clotting problems. Stomach ulcers can potentially be prevented with medications that protect the stomach lining.

There is a new generation of selective NSAIDs that cause fewer side effects. These are suxibuzone (Danilon™) and firocoxib (Equioxx™). In particular, stomach problems occur less frequently with their use.

A disadvantage of any type of painkiller is that a horse, because it feels less pain, can move more or differently than is good for it. In the case of laminitis, this is not convenient. The lamellar connection is already affected and can be further damaged by overloading.

Against the disadvantages, pain causes higher ACTH levels. Moreover, pain relief can help to take the edge off the pain, so that a laminitic horse dares to move. This is good for blood flow to its affected hooves. For a horse with EMS/ID, movement increases insulin sensitivity and helps with weight loss.

Remember that NSAIDs do not cure anything. Too much focus on the pain and its suppression can distract from the cause of the pain. An inflammation is also not a disease, but a reaction of the body.

Of course, the balance must always be struck between what is 'humane' and what is 'good' for the horse. It is a difficult choice, but you often cannot avoid it. It is not inherently good or bad to use pain-relieving medications. There is no ready-made solution for this. Discuss this topic well with your veterinarian.

ANTICOAGULANT DRUGS
In cases of laminitis, the vet may prescribe anticoagulant drugs for dissolving blood clots. These clots could result from issues like digestive problems, sudden dietary changes, or the presence of toxins in the blood. Importantly, these three issues are not directly associated with PPID.

CORTICOSTEROIDS
Medicinal corticosteroids are synthetic versions of cortisol. They are applied to tackle inflammation and infections. Like the body's own cortisol, it results in a rise in blood sugar levels. This is because corticosteroids reduce insulin sensitivity. If this is the case for a prolonged period, it can in turn cause or contribute to insulin resistance.

Corticosteroids also have a vasoconstrictive effect and they can weaken the basement membrane (see page 52). You don't want that in a horse with laminitis.

ANTIDIABETIC DRUGS
While the irreversible nature of PPID easily justifies the use of medication, this is much less the case in the treatment of insulin resistance. There is a risk that antidiabetic drug treatment is seen as an easier alternative to improving living conditions in terms of nutrition, housing, and exercise.

If you're sure you've done everything you can and you still can't get the insulin resistance under control, for example because your horse is in too much pain to exercise, then you might want to seek help in these kinds of medications.

From human medicine, substances are known that are used in the treatment of type 2 diabetes, which also have an effect on insulin-resistant horses. These are metformin and pioglitazone.

Metformin inhibits the formation of glucose from proteins and fats in the liver. In addition, it promotes the uptake of glucose by muscle cells. The drug inhibits the absorption of glucose in the small intestine. Due to these effects, there is a better regulated blood sugar level, which has a beneficial effect on both the body's sensitivity to insulin and the body weight of the horse.

However, a study from 2011 found no measurable positive effect on insulin sensitivity in ponies with insulin resistance [73]. It should be noted that the sample size was small and the ponies were not overweight.

Metformin is poorly absorbed in the horse's body. This could be an explanation for the lack of improvement in insulin sensitivity [192].

Pioglitazone is another drug that increases insulin sensitivity and has been tested for use in horses [88]. The outcomes of scientific research still leave much to be desired. Moreover, the drug appears to be carcinogenic.

THYROID HORMONES

Levothyroxine is a synthetic thyroid hormone that, when given in high doses, increases thyroid function. This accelerates metabolism, resulting in weight loss [87]. There are studies showing that sensitivity to insulin also increases [90].

Contrary to previous belief, impaired thyroid function does not play a role in EMS [114].

Unquestionably, dietary modifications and exercise are by far the preferred means of combating obesity. Nevertheless, there are cases where this remedy has merit. A PPID-afflicted horse that needs to lose weight, but is unable to move due to pain, could benefit from this remedy as a bridging measure.

OTHER DRUGS

In the fight against laminitis, the vet may further want to employ nerve-blocking, blood vessel dilating, blood pressure lowering or antihistamine drugs. It is beyond the scope of this book to discuss these.

PHYTOTHERAPY

In phytotherapy, plant-based remedies are used. However, it's important to note that herbs are not necessarily safer than chemical substances. Moreover, dosing in phytotherapy is a tricky point. You can't say for sure how large the content and biological activity of an active substance in a plant are. Another point of attention is that the active substance cannot be administered in isolation. A plant always contains other substances that you unintentionally administer. Finally, there can be an interaction with the medicines your horse gets. So, don't go therapeutic with plants and herbs at random yourself, but ask your veterinarian or a phytotherapist for advice.

There are various phytotherapeutic supplements that claim improved insulin sensitivity, a reduction in ACTH levels, an antioxidant effect, or in other ways a therapeutic advantage for horses with PPID. Conclusive and solid evidence of effectiveness in PPID-affected horses is scarce. Anticipating convincing scientific conclusions, you can still give most of these kinds of plants in consultation with a phytotherapist. They are usually quite harmless and the active substances are quickly worked out of the body. If you trust that they can replace pergolide to lower ACTH levels, you take a risk of under-treatment. Not recommended, therefore.

On the other hand, it's also not the case that a lack of evidence is the same as a lack of effectiveness. In the scientific world, there is not always an eagerness to investigate the efficacy of plants. After all, one cannot patent them. Therefore, funding for the research often falls short. Pharmaceutical companies are more interested in seeing if they can isolate the active substance to then sell it in the form of a pill or powder.

If research is then carried out, the outcomes can be biased in various ways. It goes too far in the context of this book to go into this in more depth. In summary, we can say that you should have a healthy critical attitude towards any remedy you give your horse. Seek information, ask the opinion of both proponents and opponents. Preferably from people who deal with it professionally.

Let's, after this considerable preamble, take a look at a few commonly used phytotherapeutic remedies.

CHASTEBERRY

We come across a lot of information about chasteberry (also: Vitex agnus-castus or monk's pepper) as an herb in the treatment of PPID. It contains active ingredients that could mimic some dopaminergic effects of pergolide. Scientific studies contradict each other on whether this plant helps or not.

Some studies show positive effects with regard to coat problems, sweating, polyuria/polydipsia [92]. Reduction of adiposity and less apathy are also mentioned [249]. Other studies show that these positive effects do not exist. There is even research where the clinical signs worsened in almost all examined horses [35]. In all studies, it was mainly in the early stage of PPID that positive effects were seen. For horses with advanced PPID, chasteberry is probably too little, too late.

A study was done in rats, where a high dosage of chasteberry showed an inhibitory effect on the production of prolactin by the pituitary gland [8]. On page 38 (Inappropriate milk production) you read that this hormone is produced in the anterior lobe and that there would be a connection between PPID and deregulation of the anterior lobe.

Chasteberry has no proven effect on the amount of ACTH in the blood of horses with PPID [35]. There is an unpublished study where 12 of the 25 horses had lower ACTH levels. In nine others, ACTH actually increased [165]. A lower chance of laminitis has also not been conclusively demonstrated.

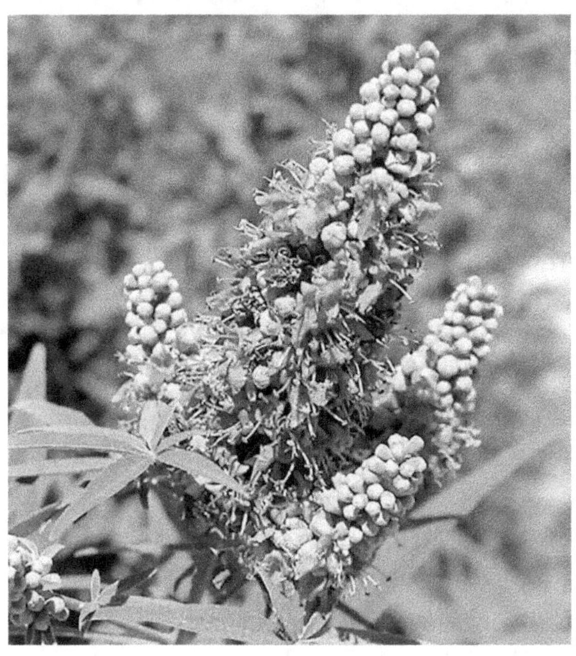

Chasteberry
(photo: Jiří Novák)

It is unclear why chasteberry does not have the effect on the intermediate lobe of the pituitary gland that we would like to see. Based on what we know about the dopaminergic effect of the active substance on the anterior lobe of the pituitary gland, it would be expected. It could be that the nerve cells in the intermediate lobe are less sensitive to the substance than those in the anterior lobe, although this has not yet been demonstrated.

Speaking of the anterior lobe: from human medicine, we know that chasteberry has an inhibitory effect on dopamine at a low dosage, while this is not the case at a high dose [75].

Whether this is also the case in horses and whether this very undesirable effect for PPID-affected equines also occurs in the intermediate lobe of the pituitary gland, we do not yet know.

Thus, chasteberry is not a serious alternative to pergolide. Because of the positive experiences reported by horse owners, it may be worth using it as supportive therapy. If you use it instead of pergolide, you take a real risk of not giving your horse the treatment it needs.

There is very little known about the combined use of chasteberry and pergolide. So, also not whether this will turn out good, neutral or bad for your horse. With regard to Parkinson's disease in humans, the combination of chasteberry with a dopamine agonist is discouraged. Always tell your vet if you want to give chasteberry alongside pergolide. Keep a close eye on blood values and changes in the clinical picture together.

A German study did see a stronger improvement in coat problems with combined use of the plant and the pill, but the ACTH levels were higher in that case than with the use of only pergolide or only chasteberry [249]. This could be because both substances act on the same receptors and get in each other's way.

To be fair, it must be said that there may simply have been too little research done. The little research that has been done was mainly carried out on rats and saw effects on hormones originating from the anterior lobe of the pituitary gland. Unfortunately, we don't have much use for that in the context of PPID.

The improvements in clinical signs could be the result of a different action of chasteberry than the supposed direct reduction of ACTH. If the improvement in the clinical picture leads to less stress and less pain, then that could lead to lower ACTH levels. Furthermore, chasteberry already has an analgesic effect. In this way, the plant might indirectly provide a better blood picture. It is tempting to adjust the dosage of pergolide based on this. Just don't forget that the ACTH that goes down due to less stress and pain comes from the anterior lobe of the pituitary gland. Reducing pergolide then means less synthetic inhibition of the intermediate lobe and thus possibly less inhibition of pituitary enlargement and formation of adenomas.

If you only start with pergolide when you can no longer suppress the clinical signs with chasteberry alone, a higher dosage is usually needed and it takes longer to get the ACTH levels under control.

TURMERIC

Turmeric is a powder made from the root of the Curcuma longa plant. Turmeric contains between 2 and 5% curcumin. This substance has an anti-inflammatory effect in rats and humans and is a potent antioxidant [82]. It also exists in the form of oil and tincture.

> **ANTIOXIDANT**
> A substance that reduces the oxidation of cells by free radicals.

Turmeric is often given to horses with EMS/insulin dysregulation. Curcumin increases the production of adiponectin [64]. Scientific sources contradict each other regarding improvements in glucose reduction and insulin resistance [82, 81]. Moreover, the studies have mainly been conducted on rats and humans.

Research has shown that curcumin in rats has an inhibitory effect on hypertrophy of cells in the anterior lobe of the pituitary gland and on hormone production in that part of the pituitary [43]. Let's hope future research shows that we can extend the line to horses and the intermediate lobe of the pituitary.

Curcumin is poorly absorbed from the small intestine and its bioavailability seems to be limited due to rapid breakdown in the liver. Piperine, a substance found in black pepper, is known to increase the bioavailability of curcumin in humans. Whether this is also the case in horses is not sufficiently known.

Despite the somewhat negative tone of this story, the trend in scientific literature is positive and hopeful that turmeric could be a good therapeutic tool. In the context of PPID, it is particularly the application in the neurodegenerative disease of Alzheimer's in humans that we should follow with attention.

MUCUNA PRURIENS

Mucuna pruriens (also: velvet bean) contains substances that may have nerve-protective effects and help increase dopamine levels in humans; particularly in those with Parkinson's disease [176]. In horses with PPID, none of this has yet been demonstrated.

GINKGO BILOBA, OREGANO

Some studies show that supplementation with ginkgo biloba (also: Japanese walnut) increases dopamine levels in rats in the long term. The same goes for oregano in mice. Again, a horse is not a rodent. As it always says so nicely at the end of many scientific articles: further research is needed to conclude whether these supplements could be successfully applied to remedy dopamine deficiency in horses with PPID.

ANTIOXIDANTS

There are plants that can have antioxidant effects. Examples of these plants are cinnamon, ginger, milk thistle, garlic, echinacea, yucca and the above discussed turmeric and ginkgo biloba. You can often find the names on the ingredient list of herbal blends sold for horses with PPID.

PSYLLIUM

Research has shown that horses given psyllium (also: fleawort) as a dietary supplement for 60 days had lower average blood sugar and insulin levels. Lower spikes in both blood sugar and insulin levels were measured, after consuming high-sugar food [220]. Horses with both PPID and insulin resistance could benefit from preventive supplementation with psyllium because of this effect. For completeness, it should be mentioned that the studies were conducted on healthy horses, i.e. without insulin resistance.

CINNAMON

Cinnamon, even at low doses, has been shown to have a beneficial effect on blood sugar levels in people with type 2 diabetes [162]. Little research has yet been done on its efficacy in horses with insulin resistance. In a 2011 study, no significant increase in insulin sensitivity was observed [159].

FENUGREEK

The seeds of fenugreek contain the amino acid 4-hydroxyleucine, which stimulates the production of insulin and increases sensitivity to this hormone. Glucose absorption is also reduced by fenugreek. Moreover, the active substances from the plant have anti-inflammatory properties [2].

MILK THISTLE

Many herbal mixtures sold ready-made for PPID horses contain seeds of milk thistle (also: St. Mary's thistle or wild artichoke). The seeds contain silymarin; a compound of which silybin is the main component. In mice, ACTH production in the anterior lobe of the pituitary gland is lowered by this substance. Cortisol production in the adrenal glands also decreases as a result [42]. Should this also be the case in horses, it would be beneficial for PPID-affected horses with hypercortisolaemia. Furthermore, silymarin has antioxidant activity.

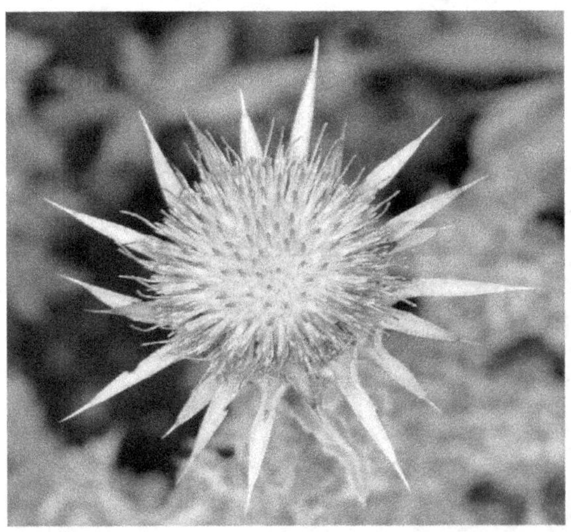

WILLOW

You can provide your horse with willow branches as a natural painkiller, specifically from almond willow or white willow, as they contain salicin. The horse can chew on the bark freely. However, excessive salicin can be harsh on the stomach, so avoid giving too much.

DEVIL'S CLAW

Devil's claw serves as an herbal substitute for NSAIDs, offering relief without the stomach-related issues associated with phenylbutazone in particular. However, it's crucial to note that devil's claw should be avoided for pregnant mares due to its abortive properties.

ANTI-INFLAMMATORIES

White willow, meadowsweet, hawthorn, devil's claw and fenugreek have anti-inflammatory effects.

ANTIOXIDANTS

In a test tube, we can measure whether a substance acts as an antioxidant, but that doesn't always mean it will have the same function in the body. Studies within human medicine on the effectiveness of antioxidant therapies have yielded mixed results. While supplementation has sometimes been shown to improve antioxidant capacity, it's not certain whether this actually provides a clinical benefit [11, 186].

Milk thistle
(photo: Vladimír Motyčka)

In horses, research has mainly focused on the therapeutic application of antioxidants in oxidative stress resulting from intense exercise, reperfusion injury (tissue damage due to renewed blood flow after oxygen shortage), and chronic respiratory problems. The various antioxidants that could potentially play a positive role in this context are vitamins A, B, C, and E, selenium, copper, zinc, superoxide dismutase (SOD), dimethyl sulfoxide (DMSO), dimethylglycine (DMG), methylsulfonylmethane (MSM), methionine, and resveratrol.

Let's not forget that in horses with PPID, there is little or no systemic oxidative stress. Whether the action of therapeutically applied antioxidants extends to the intermediate lobe of the pituitary, where oxidative stress has been demonstrated, is not yet sufficiently proven. This also applies to the plants with antioxidant action that we just discussed.

For now, the best approach seems to be to ensure healthy, natural, and varied nutrition that provides the necessary nutrients, including substances that could have an antioxidant effect.

Because vitamin E supplements are generally safe, they are often given to horses aged fifteen years or older for their antioxidant action to help prevent the development of PPID.

Again, whether this has the desired effect is still a question. Moreover, a horse that can graze a lot naturally gets enough vitamin E. In hay, the amount of this vitamin decreases. Therefore, for EMS horses on a roughage diet, it may be necessary to give a vitamin E supplement.

NUTRITION

Nutrition is an important part of living conditions to keep an eye on. It is one of the few aspects you can have complete control over.

Abrupt dietary adjustments are rarely necessary. Implement changes gradually and introduce new feed or supplements gradually over a period of four weeks. The same applies to adjustments in the quantity of food. If your horse is laminitic, it may be necessary to modify the diet more quickly, especially when the horse is getting food that is high in sugar and starch.

HORMONAL DYSREGULATION

PPID is primarily a neurological problem, but the total hormonal dysregulation that results from it is what the horse suffers from. You have seen all kinds of hormones pass by, starting with those produced in the pituitary gland. Then we discussed insulin, leptin, adiponectin, cortisol, and a whole host of other hormones. Things can go wrong with all these hormones. The interaction between them makes it all a bit more complicated. Moreover, hormonal dysregulation is never a black-and-white issue. Cortisol dysregulation, in particular (see page 24), is more complex than often thought. This also applies to EMS/insulin dysregulation.

It would be a bit naive to think that there are horses with PPID that can continue eating the way they did when they were hormonally fine. That is why it is best to feed every PPID horse as an 'insulin resistance risk horse'. Even if they are not overweight; even if they have never had laminitis.

Take advantage of the fact that there are equine nutritionists who are happy to help you scrutinise your horse's diet and tailor it specifically to its situation and needs.

MUSCLE ATROPHY

As muscle atrophy (muscle loss) is both a clinical manifestation of PPID and a normal feature of ageing, we will discuss the special nutritional needs of horses affected by this when discussing seniors.

WEIGHT MANAGEMENT

There are horses with PPID who are either overweight or underweight, with or without insulin dysregulation. For all these horses, the focus should be on a diet that enables them to regain or maintain their ideal body condition.

Overweight should be combated with dietary adjustments and physical exercise. For horses that are too thin, dietary adjustments should aim at a healthy and controlled weight gain.

SUPPLEMENTS

Of certain minerals, vitamins and trace elements your horse needs a minimum amount. In particular, horses eating mainly hay or on a diet for weight loss are more likely to have deficiencies than horses that are put out to pasture unrestrictedly.

ROUGHAGE ANALYSIS

Before you start giving supplements, you first need to know which vitamins, minerals, trace elements, and the like your horse is lacking. A blood test can help with this, although this is not 100% reliable for all values. Therefore, important information is obtained from a roughage analysis. If you know what your horse is getting too little of through its diet, you know what you need to supplement.

Starting from £20 ($25), you can have roughage tested for energy, sugars, proteins, and dry matter content.
A more comprehensive forage analysis, covering a wide range of essential nutrients, will typically cost more than a basic analysis. The cost can depend on the number and types of nutrients being analysed, as well as the specific laboratory conducting the analysis. For a thorough analysis that includes multiple essential nutrients such as minerals, vitamins, and additional parameters, the cost per sample can range from £50 to £150 in the UK ($60-$180 in the US). Armed with this information, a nutrition expert can precisely recommend supplements. In the meantime, you can use a 'balancer,' which includes vital vitamins, minerals, and trace elements.

> ## BALANCER
>
> A broad-spectrum supplement, often referred to as a balancer, is designed to harmonise a forage ration by providing the necessary daily amounts of vitamins, minerals, and trace elements.
>
> A balancer is second to a supplement formulated by a nutritionist specifically for your horse based on forage analysis and possibly blood test results.
>
> Read the ingredient list thoroughly. Certain balancers may contain nearly 20% sugar and starch.
>
> If your horse is already receiving a balancer, there's no need to provide additional minerals through its lick. A simple salt lick is sufficient.

Compile your hay sample from small tufts from different bales that come from the same land and were cut at the same time. When you have hay from different batches, it is best to have each batch analysed separately. If you have small quantities from different batches, an analysis is of little use and it is better to assume average values of hay.

SOIL ANALYSIS

Consider having a soil sample analysed as well, as minerals absent in the soil won't magically appear in the grass. It's important to note that the results of a soil analysis may not accurately represent the minerals eventually absorbed by the grass plant. However, such an analysis serves as a solid foundation for fertiliser recommendations.

DRINKING WATER

Water is by far the most important nutrient, but is least often seen as such. In the case of polyuria/polydipsia and hypohidrosis, drinking water supply is extra important. Read more about drinking water in the sidebar on the next page.

PROTEINS AND AMINO ACIDS

Apart from the horse's overall protein intake, its quality must also be high. This means that the proteins must provide enough essential amino acids. Essential amino acids are those that the horse cannot produce (synthesise) and must obtain through its diet. While this is generally not an issue, special attention is needed for methionine, lysine, and threonine.

VITAMINS

For vitamins, it is also true that the horse can make some of them itself, especially B1, B6 and B12, C and K, while others must be in the diet.

As horses get older, they are less able to synthesise certain vitamins themselves. This is particularly the case with B vitamins and vitamin C.

Old horses with PPID, even in the subclinical stage, have lower blood vitamin C levels than healthy or younger horses [173]. Supplementation may be necessary.

Especially when horses with PPID get no or less access to pasture, supplementation of vitamin C and E is recommended. Grass is a good source of these vitamins, but when the grass is cut and dried, the levels decrease considerably.

A study conducted in 2020 discovered reduced levels of vitamin B12 in horses with PPID, irrespective of their age [227]. Vitamin B12 is crucial for the optimal functioning of the brain and nervous system. In humans, deficiency in B12 has been linked to conditions such as Parkinson's disease [252].

DRINKING WATER

Opt for tap water as it is the safest water source for your horse. Ensure it remains consistently fresh. Maintain the drinking water supply by preventing the presence of algae, dead leaves, insects, manure, urine, and rust. In winter, take precautions to prevent freezing.

If giving tap water is not possible, alternative water sources exist, but they come with drawbacks. Pumped groundwater (well water), rainwater, and surface water may carry contaminants. Consider testing the water for potential contamination.

Also keep an eye on the quality of your rainwater. Zinc roof boards, gutters, and downspouts can increase the water's zinc content significantly.

Stagnant and other surface water can be polluted by illegal discharges, manure, pesticides, and may harbour blue-green algae and salmonella. It is the least favourable choice for providing water to your horse.

People suffering from Cushing's disease have also been found to be frequently deficient in B12 [240]. It is important to note that these findings in humans do not necessarily imply that this line can be extended to horses with PPID.

MINERALS AND TRACE ELEMENTS

Minerals and trace elements need to be absorbed in specific ratios, as an imbalanced ratio can lead to an excess of one mineral impeding the absorption of another.

Furthermore, an excessive abundance of certain vitamins or minerals can be as detrimental as a deficiency.

Salt lick

Sodium is a mineral that horses may struggle to obtain in adequate quantities. Among other things, it is important for transmitting stimuli within the nervous system. Provide a plain, white salt lick without additional minerals or trace elements. Avoid flavoured stones with apple or molasses. The horse should lick the stone for salt intake, not due to taste preference. Be cautious with red-coloured stones, as they often contain excessive amounts of iron.

Zinc, selenium, copper and iron

The minerals zinc, selenium and copper are almost always too low in roughage. This is because they are already too low in the soil. In contrast, iron levels are often far too high. This makes the absorption of zinc, selenium and copper even more difficult. On page 42 you read that there is a link between iron excess and insulin resistance.

Omega fatty acids

Maintaining the right ratio of omega fatty acids is important to prevent a pro-inflammatory property of a particular fatty acid from taking over. Horses that consume little or no fresh grass may lack omega-3 fatty acids in their diet, making supplementation advisable. Good sources of omega-3 fatty acids include flaxseed and cold-pressed flaxseed oil.

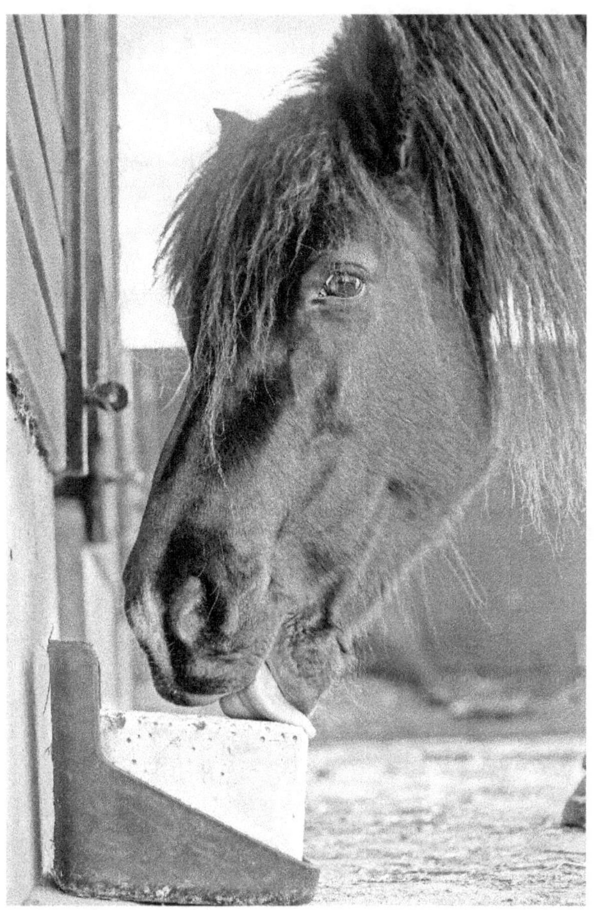

Simple white salt lick
(photo: Karin Schouwenburg)

Pasture or not?

Reading this, you will understand that it is beyond the scope of this book to go into all the details here. The basis of a healthy ration is roughage. If the horse has pasture access, it is important to take into account the amount of sugar present in the grass. Grazing on a pasture is still possible for many horses with PPID, but it is advisable to adjust your grazing policy.

Not all grasses produce the same amount of sugars. A varied pasture with many species that produce less sugars is more than desirable. Furthermore, it is advisable not to put horses out to pasture during April and May when sugar levels are often high, and during the seasonal rise.

For PPID horses that are not insulin-resistant, limited grazing should be possible in the remaining months, provided ACTH is under control and they are not overweight. Signs of laminitis are also a no-go. In the sidebars on the page opposite, read how you can gain even more control over food intake and sugar consumption with well-chosen grazing times and restrictions.

HAY
The safest thing to do is to make the ration of your horse with PPID consist mostly of hay; even in summer. Ensure that the hay has a combined sugar and starch content of less than 10%. Since grasses in the United Kingdom and the majority of the USA typically do not store starch, attention should primarily be focused on monitoring the sugar content in practice.

The Midwestern United States, Australia and New Zealand do have grasses that convert sugar into starch instead of fructan.

If there are still grass seeds present in the hay, keep in mind that these do contain a significant amount of starch. So, don't let your PPID horse eat the 'grit' left at the bottom of the wheelbarrow, as it mainly consists of grass seeds.

If your horse is at an optimal weight and solely fed on roughage other than grass, provide it with approximately 1.5% to 2% of its weight in dry matter (DM, see page 118) over a 24-hour period. For example, for a 600-kilo (1320 lbs) horse, this equates to a daily intake of 6 to 8 kg (13.2 to 17.6 lbs) of dry matter.

Dry, unpacked hay usually contains 85-90% DM. So, you give between 10 and 14 kilos (22-31 lbs) of this per 24 hours, depending on the horse's body weight. If it is too fat, give less; if it is too thin, give more. If it already consumes 2% of its body weight in DM and is still too thin, you can add more hay. Most horses will eat up to about 2.5% of their body weight in DM; pony breeds usually eat even more.

What also matters is the type of roughage. Here again, a roughage analysis provides clarity. In general, hard, stalky hay has a lower energy value (contains fewer calories) than softer, finer hay. For an overweight PPID horse or one prone to easy weight gain, that coarse-stemmed hay is preferable.

Continue on page 118

WHEN IS PASTURE GRASS THE SAFEST?

The rule of thumb is that grass sugar levels are lowest at night and in the very early morning, when the temperature has not dropped below 5 °C (41 °F) at night, while sufficient water and nutrients were available, and the grass plant predominantly has leaves and no heads.

During the day, sugar levels will rise. More hours of sunshine result in higher sugar content. As spring progresses, this will become more and more the case. Cloud cover and shade, however, decelerate this rise.

Monitor not only the sugar content but also the overall quantity of grass your horse consumes. In spring grass growth is rapid. Even if a horse ingests a large amount of grass with a low sugar percentage, it can still consume too much sugar. In such situations or if you suspect excessive sugar in the grass, implement measures to restrict grazing.

RESTRICT GRAZING

To prevent your PPID-affected horse, without insulin resistance and with well-managed ACTH levels, from eating too much or too fast and thus taking in too many carbohydrates on pasture, you can adopt the following measures to restrict grazing:

- Use a grazing muzzle. Grass leaf tips contain less sugar. A grazing muzzle attached to the halter helps prevent the horse from grazing lower grass portions. Grazing speed decreases and food enters the digestive tract more slowly and steadily. In this way the digestion can take place more slowly and effectively. What's more, your horse can stay out on pasture longer and therefore will get more exercise. Ensure the muzzle fits well and allows your horse to drink normally.
- Prevent overgrazing, as the shorter nibbled grass contains a lot of sugars. Implement strip grazing by shifting, enlarging, or reducing the grazing area daily using electric fencing and stakes.
- Divide your field into plots and allow your horse to graze a plot until the grass is about 4 centimetres (1 ½ inch) high. Then move the horse to the next plot, allowing the grazed area to regrow.

Merely restricting the horse's time in the pasture is insufficient. In 2011, a study was conducted on the amount of grass and hay that ponies eat when they are restricted in their grazing time. The striking results of this study were that in the first week of observation, per daily three-hour grazing session, the ponies consumed an amount equivalent to about half a per cent of their body weight. By week six, this had doubled to almost one per cent. The study showed that, over six weeks, the animals learned the importance of moving on when put out to pasture [22].

DRY MATTER

Dry matter is what remains of feed plants after they are completely dried. The higher the moisture content of the food, the lower the dry matter content.

Horses need a daily intake of 1.5 to 2.5% of their body weight in dry matter. From food with a low dry matter content, they must consume larger quantities to meet this requirement. However, if this food is rich in energy (calories), it may be detrimental for a horse aiming to shed excess weight. An instance of such calorie-dense consumption is extensive grazing during the spring and summer.

A roughage analysis will provide information on the dry matter content.

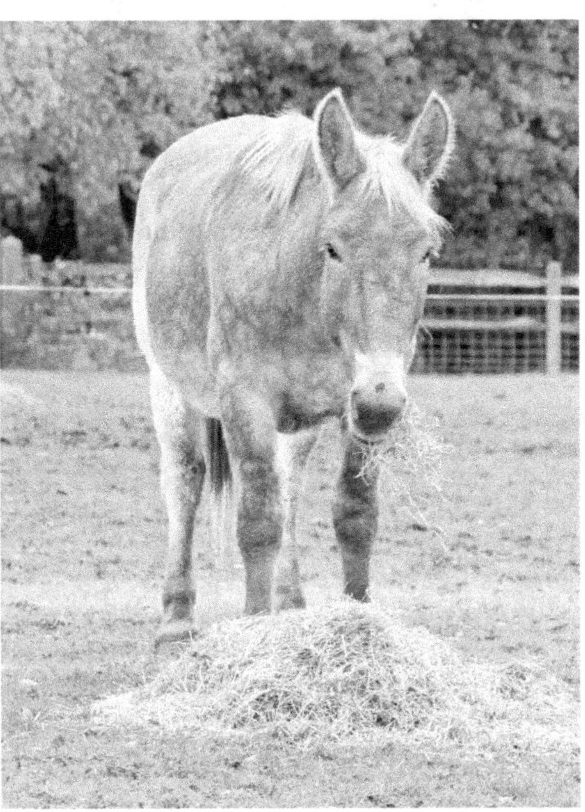

(photo: Mulography)

On the other hand, if the horse tends to lose weight easily and struggles to maintain good weight, a softer, finer hay with a higher energy value is better. In both cases, it is important that the hay has a low sugar content.

CONCENTRATES

Pellets, concentrates and cereals are not a good idea. These foods typically contain excessive quick sugars and starches and are often fed in portions, leading to significant spikes in blood sugar levels. The digestive system of a horse, a natural grazer, is not well-suited for this type of feeding.

Horse muesli is essentially pellets before being ground and pressed. Opt for muesli without grains, which stays below 10% in sugar and starch content. An occasional handful of this variant poses no harm. However, some brands of muesli can exceed 20%, so it's advisable to refrain from purchasing those.

If you do want to feed concentrates, read the label very carefully. Go for low sugar and starch. Cereals should also be avoided. Also pay attention to the amount of iron in the product. This should be as low as possible. For old horses or horses that are in poor condition (lean, muscle atrophy), you will want to see the ingredients, vitamins and minerals we list separately in the following paragraphs.

Be cautious with product names containing 'Cush' or 'Senior.' Some of these products may contain over 20% sugars and starches, despite their seemingly targeted names.

SENIORS

Not every horse with PPID necessarily has EMS/ID or is overweight; some may actually struggle to maintain weight. For these horses, a tailored nutritional approach is necessary, aiming for a healthy and gradual weight gain without resorting to sugary and starchy foods. PPID is more prevalent in older horses, and they are often prone to being underweight due to the natural aging process or dental issues.

GUTS

Nutrient absorption predominantly takes place in the small intestine, and this process becomes less efficient in older horses. Consequently, older horses often need to consume more food than when they were younger to maintain their weight.

As horses age, the large intestine (colon) may experience a decline in its ability to digest fibre effectively. This could be attributed to alterations in the gut's microbiome. Additionally, reduced chewing ability in older horses may contribute to the entry of larger fibres into the intestines.

MICROBIOME
Community of micro-organisms, including bacteria, unicellular organisms, yeasts, parasites, and viruses, that inhabit various parts of the body, such as the intestines.

Old horses may struggle to digest very coarse-stemmed hay effectively. In contrast, soaked grass pellets, soaked beet pulp, and soya hulls tend to digest well. Additionally, considering the decline in B vitamin production in the colon mentioned earlier, supplementation may become necessary for older horses.

Whereas a balancer is fairly harmless, you should not experiment at random with supplementing loose vitamins and minerals. Ask an equine nutritionist for advice.

ALFALFA HAY

Alfalfa hay (or lucerne) is rich in easily digestible fibres and contains approximately 20% easily digestible protein, aiding in reducing muscle breakdown. However, it may have an excess of calcium, which can be detrimental to the kidneys and impact phosphorus availability. One solution is to mix it with hay that has lower calcium content to achieve a balanced ratio.

Alfalfa hay is also a source of crucial amino acids such as methionine, lysine, and threonine, and it is abundant in magnesium. Another protein-rich plant from the same family as alfalfa is esparcette.

Older horses more often have difficulty digesting proteins properly in the small intestine. Once again, alfalfa hay and soya hulls stand out as effective options. They provide high-quality proteins that you can feed to meet protein needs without overfeeding your horse. For horses with muscle atrophy, proteins and the essential amino acids they provide are also very important to build muscle mass.

Supplementing high-quality amino acids frequently proves effective in maintaining muscle mass and preventing muscle atrophy in older horses.

FEEDING PRACTICE

Older, weaker horses may face challenges at feeding spots due to interactions with herd mates. Additionally, those with dental issues may require more time to eat. In both cases, it's advisable to feed them separately, allowing for closer monitoring of food intake and reducing stress. Alternatively, spreading roughage in multiple locations can be a practical solution.

DCP

To get a more accurate indication of the protein requirement of a horse, the amount of digestible crude protein (DCP) is used. This is the total amount of protein in the feed that the horse can actually digest.

The daily basic requirement of DCP for an adult horse of 600 kg (1325 lbs), that does not work, is about 0.6 grams (0.02 oz) per kg of body weight. For lighter horses, that number is higher, for heavier horses lower.

This basic requirement is no more than a starting point. Breed, age, body weight, the way the horse is kept and the amount of work are all variables. There can also be individual differences between horses. Ask your nutritionist or veterinarian for an estimate of the amount of DCP that your senior needs.

Older horses are more prone to osteoarthritis, which can make eating from ground level or pulling hay from a net painful. Help these horses find a place to eat peacefully and pain-free.

When offering soaked food, be mindful of potential fermentation in summer and freezing in winter. To prevent bacterial and fungal growth, provide an amount that the horse can consume in one meal, which may require feeding several times a day.

TEETH

Grazing becomes challenging when the front teeth (incisors) are missing or crooked in the mouth and upper and lower jaw teeth do not connect properly when the horse's head is at ground level. In such cases, providing good hay or grass fodder remains suitable as long as the molars are in good condition. Ask your equine dentist if they can help address specific dental concerns.

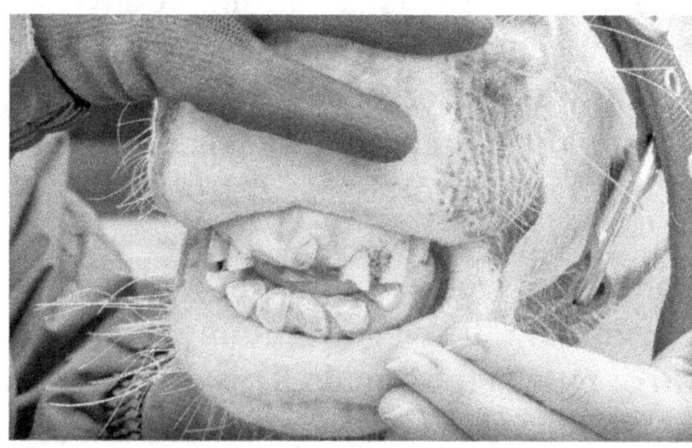

Grazing no longer goes well with these teeth

(photo: Redwings Horse Sanctuary)

With worn or damaged molars, grinding food is more difficult. Old horses with bad teeth cannot chew hay enough to swallow and digest it properly. Grass usually still goes fine for these horses, but is only an option when it is safe and there is no increased risk of laminitis. Switching from coarse, stalky hay to fine, soft hay is the next step. When they can no longer eat that well either, you can give a roughage substitute with short stalks. If that too is no longer possible, the next step is soaked grass chunks. Most old horses can still eat

this for a long time. You could possibly supplement this with some grain-free mash or soaked beet pulp (see sidebar on the next page).

UNDERWEIGHT HORSES

Because of the pot belly and adiposity, it might sometimes not immediately be noticeable that the horse is losing weight and muscles are breaking down. Because horses with PPID are often older, weight loss is also more often seen as inevitable. As a result, underweight horses more often go unnoticed. If the horse was previously too fat and diet and exercise programmes have been pursued a little too fanatically, there is a danger that it will now actually become too thin, without you as the owner noticing. Ask your equine nutritionist or vet to evaluate and discuss your horse's weight and overall condition.

We discuss underweight horses with PPID here. There are a variety of other possible causes of weight loss, some of which may lead to irreparable damage or prove fatal. When in the slightest doubt about the cause of emaciation, always ask your vet for advice. Obviously, you have already ruled out or addressed worm infestation, dental problems and stomach ulcers as possible causes.

Feeding recommendations for horses with PPID that need to gain weight can be tricky. Striking the right balance involves adding calories without introducing excessive amounts of sugar and starch into their diet.

FAT AND OIL

To add more calories, people do feed high-fat foods. Feeding large amounts of oil or other fat can exacerbate or even trigger insulin resistance. It is therefore important to use a balanced combination of fats and carbohydrates to promote weight gain in lean horses with PPID with caution.

Too-lean horses with insulin dysregulation may benefit from soaked beet pulp, soya hulls or (chopped) alfalfa hay, combined with vegetable oils that are low in omega-6 fatty acids (e.g. linseed or rapeseed oil). This allows you to feed energy-rich feed without risking causing strong insulin spikes. This is because these feeds contain a lot of slowly digestible dietary fibre (structural carbohydrates). Flaxseed is rich in fats that are good for your horse. Depending on the amount of supplementary feed, give this divided into several portions per day.

Some oils, such as sunflower and corn oil, contain the wrong amount and ratio of omega fatty acids. This does your horse more harm than good.

BEET PULP

Beet pulp is left over from the production of sugar from sugar beets. The sugar is gone. What remains are just the easily digestible dietary fibres. These contain a lot of calories, which are released slowly. The sugar and starch content is usually low. Beet pulp is a good source of protein and the amino acids methionine, lysine and threonine.

However beet pulp does not contain sufficient vitamins and is not balanced in minerals. It can be difficult to get the ratio between calcium and phosphorus right if you feed a lot of it. It also contains very few trace elements. It is very suitable as a supplement, but certainly not as the main component of the ration to replace grass and hay. It is best to consult an equine nutritionist if you want to give more than one kilo (2.2 lbs) of beet pulp per day to an older horse.

Choose quick-soaking beet pulp. This only needs to be soaked for ten minutes. Make sure that the sugar content is below 10% and preferably even lower.

Normal beet pulp must be soaked for at least twelve hours to prevent oesophageal blockages. This pulp often contains more sugar than the quick-soaking variant. Moreover, the exact sugar content is not always on the packaging. This can easily be much higher than 10%.

HAYLAGE

Haylage can serve as a suitable alternative for PPID-affected horses without insulin dysregulation who struggle with weight maintenance. Its softer texture makes it easier to chew, and it is somewhat more digestible due to the fermentation process. However, it's essential to consider the sugar and calorie content in haylage, especially if harvested early when grass was very young. Opting for haylage harvested a bit later can be a better choice.

Contrary to popular belief, haylage does not contain more sugars than hay. If you cut a field and let one half of the clippings dry to 85% DM and then bale it as hay, and you let the other half dry to 70% DM after which you wrap it in plastic, both products will initially have similar sugar content. But if you look six months later, the haylage will have a lower sugar content than the hay, due to bacterial fermentation consuming some sugars. So why haylage still sometimes has a higher sugar content is mainly a result of the time of harvest. Haylage has a lower dry matter content than hay. Therefore, you need to feed more of it.

In horses with insulin dysregulation, haylage can yield a relatively high insulin response. This would be due not so much to sugars, but to other substances, such as volatile fatty acids and ethanol [158].

Grazing is also still a good way for underweight horses to gain weight. Build this up slowly. Do not let your PPID-afflicted horse out to pasture until ACTH is under control, when it is insulin resistant or when there are signs of laminitis.

LET THEM EAT QUIETLY

Heavily emaciated horses are less able to defend their social position and access to food. Not only do they not get enough food, but they will also eat too quickly and anxiously. As a result, they chew less well and cannot utilise nutrients as well. So, like the seniors, it is better to feed them separately.

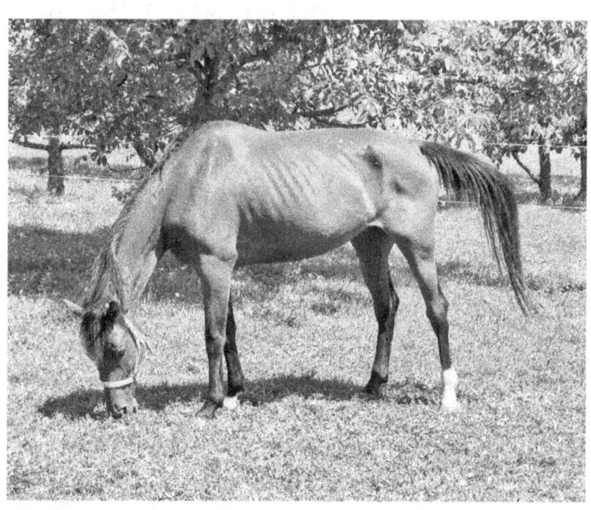

Give an underweight horse time to eat quietly
(photo: Anna Armbrust)

EMS/INSULIN DYSREGULATION AND OVERWEIGHT

Even if we do not yet know exactly how it is, it is still wise to assume that a horse with PPID has an increased risk of insulin resistance, even without being overweight. It is imperative to keep ACTH under control and to regularly have insulin and glucose levels in the blood measured in order to intervene adequately to prevent laminitis.

A large proportion of horses with PPID also have EMS/insulin dysregulation and obesity. Addressing this problem should be based on weight management and exercise. We will first look at how food adjustments can be used for weight management. Then we will talk about exercise.

For the horses discussed here, dietary adjustments are very important to see weight loss. Also, you don't want the hormonal problems associated with EMS to get worse. Ideally, the goal is not only to halt but also to reduce and eventually eliminate these problems. Notably, insulin dysregulation tends to improve as the horse loses weight.

There is a direct link between obesity and oxidative stress [152]. The rule of thumb is: less excess weight reduces oxidative stress. It is one of the keys in the fight against PPID.

We mentioned earlier that pellets and cereals are to be avoided for horses that are at a good weight. For horses that need to lose weight, this is even more so. It contains way too many sugars and starches. Nor is a horse's digestive system built for it. Large spikes in blood sugar levels will be the result. This is detrimental to horses with insulin resistance in general and to horses with EMS in particular. It only makes them fatter.

Foods high in sugars and cereals lower the amount of adiponectin in the blood. On page 44 you read that this hormone is important for keeping blood sugar levels optimal. So, a drop is not good.

An ideal diet for overweight horses involves high-fibre roughage, preferably hay, with a high dry matter content and less than 10% ethanol-soluble carbohydrates (refer to the 'Sugar types' sidebar on the next page) and starch combined in the dry matter. For horses with severe insulin resistance, it is recommended to keep the limit at 8%, with a preference for starch not exceeding 4%. This diet aims to fill the gut and provide energy in the form of volatile fatty acid.

For severely insulin-resistant horses, those prone to recurrent laminitis, and those requiring substantial weight loss, grazing is really out of the question, as grass can be more hazardous for them than other types of roughage.

SUGAR TYPES

We refer to sugars in horse food, but we should actually call them carbohydrates. That is a broader term. There are carbohydrates that are not sugar, such as fructan, starch, and dietary fibre.

We can divide carbohydrates into:
- Simple and double carbohydrates, such as glucose, fructose, and sucrose. Because these are commonly associated with rapid energy release, they are also called 'fast sugars'.
- Fructan
- Complex carbohydrates, such as starch and dietary fibre

If you have your hay analysed and read labels on horse feed, you may also come across these abbreviations for the different types of carbohydrates:

- ESC: Ethanol-Soluble Carbohydrates = simple and double carbohydrates
- WSC: Water-Soluble Carbohydrates = ESC + fructan
- NSC: Non-Structural Carbohydrates = WSC + starch
- SC: Structural Carbohydrates = dietary fibre

FRUCTAN

When there is an excess of sugar for growth, the grasses in our pastures store it as fructan, a specific type of complex carbohydrate, to use during favourable growth conditions.

It was long thought that most horses became laminitic from ingesting too much fructan. Fructan does have an impact on the onset or exacerbation of laminitis, but only in SIRS-related laminitis. We see this form of laminitis in only about 10% of all cases, and even then, it can stem from various other causes. Moreover, a horse can never ingest so much fructan while grazing that it can cause laminitis independently.

In PPID cases, horses experience endocrinopathic laminitis, where fructan has no involvement. It is the sugars and the hormonal reaction to them that cause the trouble.

Nonetheless, it is not entirely unnecessary to monitor fructan warnings through an app or fructan index online. These systems are valuable for estimating recent sugar levels in plants. Elevated fructan levels result from a previous sugar surplus, and there is a risk of recurrence in the short term, posing a danger to your PPID-afflicted horse with endocrinopathic laminitis. Moreover, the three distinct forms of laminitis (refer to page 50) can coexist. Avoid introducing potential causes of laminitis. Consider very effort to prevent laminitis as worthwhile.

The problem lies in the unpredictable variation of fast sugars in grass throughout the day and the year, making it almost impossible to control sugar and energy intake. For these horses, opting for a paddock paradise (see sidebar on page 148) or a dry paddock, along with customised nutritional advice from an equine nutritionist, is the recommended approach.

HAY

If your horse needs to lose weight, aim for your horse to get 20-30% fewer calories than it needs, to create a so-called negative energy balance. How much hay it should have depends on its energy value (calories), which a nutritionist can precisely calculate with a hay analysis.

With energy-rich (or high-calorie) hay, it is an impossible task to make your horse lose weight without compromising fibre intake. Even with energy-poor (low-calorie) hay, finding the right balance between low calories and sufficient fibre requires trial and error. Avoid crash diets, as they can 'freeze' metabolism and worsen insulin resistance.

STRAW

If your hay is a bit too rich, you can either soak it (see sidebar on the next page) or mix it with oat or barley straw (maximum 50-50) [150].

Digesting large amounts of straw forms ammonia compounds, straining the liver. Avoid going beyond a 50-50 mix of straw and hay to prevent this strain.

Mixing straw with soaked hay is also an option, but only if your horse's teeth can still chew properly. Check the fibres you find in the manure. If these are longer than 2.5 cm (1 inch), you should ask the dentist to assess the teeth and touch them up if necessary. Wheat straw has too much lignin, making it difficult for horses with bad teeth to chew easily.

Straw contains too little protein, but mixing it with alfalfa hay can restore a balanced protein content. Weight loss diets often require supplementation. Reducing hay quantity and opting for lower quality increases nutritional deficiencies in its ration.

The way the feed is offered can also sometimes be improved. With a slow feeder, the speed at which the hay is eaten can be reduced. This is better for the horse's digestion.

Some people give old hay on the assumption that this contains less sugars. This is not true. Old hay only contains less vitamins and more dust.

SOAKING HAY

If you don't have low-sugar hay, soak and rinse your hay. In just 15 minutes of rinsing, you can eliminate a substantial amount of fast sugars and fructan (water-soluble carbohydrates/ WSC) from the hay [69]. Using more or fresh water enhances this leaching process, and warm water rinses twice as fast as cold water.

Unfortunately, soaking also removes important water-soluble minerals and vitamins. Therefore, you should always give a broad-spectrum supplement (balancer) to horses that get soaked hay.

For horses with EMS who quickly become laminitic, it may be necessary to soak for a long time; up to 16 hours. Unfortunately, even long soaking does not guarantee that sufficient sugar has leeched away. According to a 2011 study, depending on the type of hay, the WSC content may still be too high [91].

Soak the hay in a large tub or wheelbarrow, then rinse and let it drain thoroughly. Needless to say: don't give the residual water to the horse to drink as that now contains the sugars.

Do not soak more hay than the horse can eat in one day. Wet hay can easily become mouldy.

Initially, your horse might not show enthusiasm, but over time, it will acclimatise to eating the soaked hay. If the reluctance persists, consider mixing it with a small amount of dry hay, gradually reducing the ratio.

When uncertain about the hay's carbohydrate content, it is safer to soak it in winter as well. The hay might have been harvested when the grass was high in sugars, which will remain present in the hay.

Beet pulp can be soaked without any problems. However, avoid soaking haylage as it may undergo a second fermentation, promoting the growth of undesirable bacteria. Since haylage already has lower WSC than hay, soaking is unnecessary.

SEED HAY

Grass seed hay is a by-product of cultivating grass for seed. The majority of non-structural carbohydrates (NSC) are concentrated in the seed, which is intended for the seed trade. The stalks primarily contain dietary fibre (structural carbohydrates) and, when dried into hay, serve as low-energy roughage suitable for horses dealing with laminitis or those requiring weight loss. Think of it as straw from a grass rather than a cereal. Grass hay is notably low in energy and has lower amounts of vitamins, minerals, trace elements, and proteins compared to richer hay.

CHOPPED FODDER

Roughage is also sold chopped. Sometimes as a single type, for example, chopped alfalfa hay, sometimes as a mixture of different types of roughage. Usually, it contains hay, alfalfa, and straw.

GRASS PELLETS

Grass pellets, whether soaked or not, are quickly eaten. This poses a risk for overweight horses as they may intake excessive sugars.

WEIGHT LOSS

Usually, weight loss goes quite well in the beginning. It then decreases after three to four months, as the metabolism adapts to the diet [255].

Make sure weight loss is gradual and not too fast. If weight loss is too rapid, there is a risk – especially in Shetland ponies, Welsh ponies, Haflingers, fjords and donkeys – of hyperlipidaemia (blood fattening).

There is also a risk of increased insulin response if weight loss is too rapid. A weight loss of 1% of target weight or 0.5% of current body weight per week, whichever number is lowest, is justified.

Monitor weight loss carefully to ensure that the objective (the target weight and the rate at which it is achieved) is met, but not exceeded.

WEIGHING HAY OR COUNTING CALORIES

There are significant individual differences in weight loss in horses put on a diet. Some shed pounds rapidly, while in others, following the same feeding regimen, it is very difficult.

Unfortunately, this difference is also largely explained by the fact that many weight loss recommendations only specify the quantity of hay to provide. The calorie intake for the horse remains undisclosed. As mentioned a few pages earlier, a nutritionist can precisely determine the suitable amount of hay for your horse, based on hay analysis.

INSULIN RESISTANCE

A direct causal link between EMS and PPID has not yet been scientifically proven, but since there is increasing thought in that direction, here one could say 'no harm no foul'. Moreover, there is a link between cortisol dysregulation and insulin resistance (IR) [135]. An anti-IR diet is therefore healthier for all horses.

As insulin resistance is directly linked to laminitis, it is also good to adjust the diet. This way, you can prevent IR from getting worse or developing, should your horse not already have it. Remember that the chronic or recurrent severe pain of laminitis is the most common reason for deciding to euthanise laminitic horses.

Autumn is a difficult period for horses with PPID. ESC is high in autumn grass, horses eat more leading up to winter, there is a stronger insulin response and there is the seasonal rise in melanocortins. So pay attention.

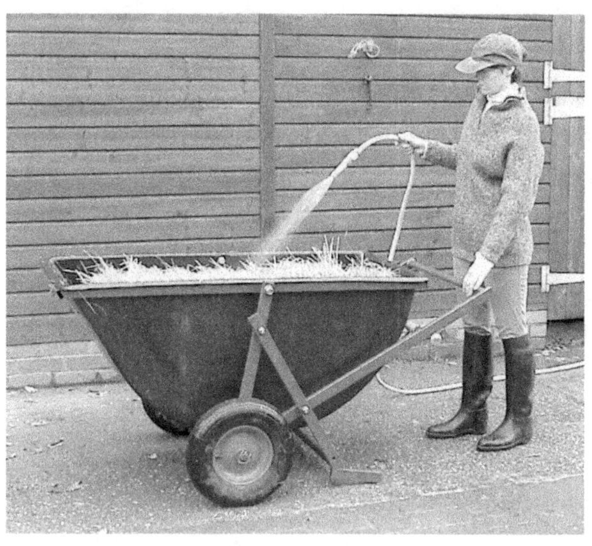

Soaking hay
(photo: Classic Equine Equipment)

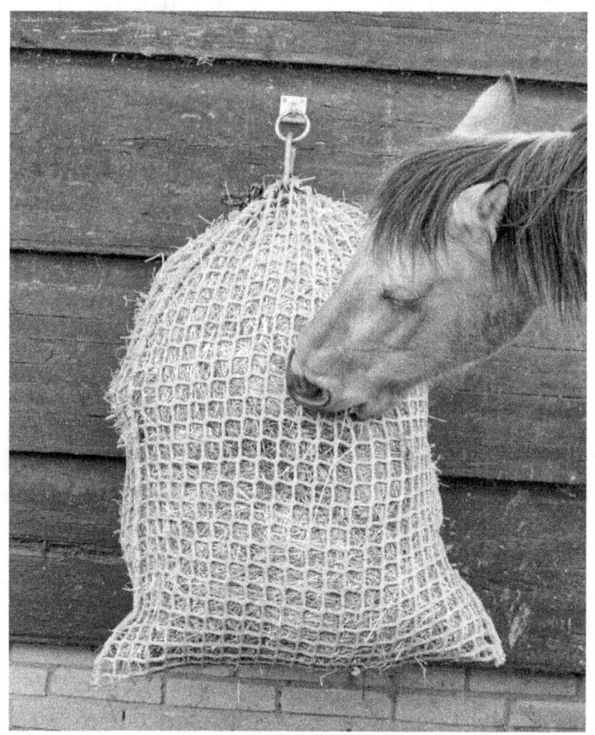

Slowfeeder haynet
(photo: Marsha Brouwer/PaardEerlijk)

Some pellets sold specifically for old horses contain more than 30% sugars and starch. This is not a good feed in general and certainly not for the overweight PPID horse with IR. Again: read the label.

Supplements

Omega-3 fatty acids obtained from microalgae may have a beneficial effect on insulin metabolism and blood triglyceride levels, and they may reduce inflammation, according to a 2019 study [84]. Another study showed that horses fed food enriched with dried microalgae lost weight and their insulin sensitivity improved [238].

Supplementation with prebiotic fibre could improve insulin sensitivity in obese horses to some extent [55]. Beet pulp contains a lot of pectin. This is one such prebiotic fibre.

As so often, for these types of supplements, you will find both studies showing efficacy and studies that cannot confirm the positive effects. Because they are generally safe to give and because there is a lot of anecdotal evidence (satisfied users) for them, you can always give them a try.

Dosage does matter when using prebiotics. In fact, they are actually fructans. In excessive amounts, they disrupt the microbiome of the colon, which could contribute to the development of SIRS-related laminitis.

MAGNESIUM AND CHROME

According to a study conducted in 2016, the mineral magnesium might enhance insulin sensitivity in horses with EMS/insulin dysregulation that do not have a magnesium deficiency [184]. However, the BCS, CNS, and body weight of the horses in this study did not decrease. A 2011 study could not demonstrate this effect [73]. The disparity in results might be attributed to the use of different magnesium compounds in the studies, namely magnesium aspartate and magnesium oxide.

A magnesium deficiency contributes to impaired carbohydrate metabolism. Research from 2020 revealed that horses with EMS/insulin dysregulation are more prone to magnesium deficiency compared to those without this metabolic condition [226].

A 2020 study suggested that chromium could enhance insulin sensitivity in healthy, non-insulin-resistant horses [23]. Note that chromium as a supplement for horses is not allowed in Europe.

SOIL, PLANTS AND THE MICROBIOME

Earlier, we talked about healthy, natural and varied food that provides the nutrients the horse needs. This actually starts with healthy soil, which provides a rich variety of plants that supply all kinds of important nutrients. These contribute to a healthy and balanced microbiome in the intestine (gut flora).

Let's first look at soil. Many different micro-organisms, insects, worms and all kinds of other life inhabit a healthy soil. This soil is neither too dry nor too wet, is well-rooted and full of nutrients. Healthy soil is free of pesticides and fertilisers.

Many different plants grow, providing the horse with important nutrients such as vitamins, minerals, trace elements and so-called polyphenols. Polyphenols are substances that play an important role in the immune system and in recovery from diseases. Some polyphenols, such as resveratrol, have antioxidant properties.

Plant species diversity also increases the amount of organic matter available to the soil. This reduces the need to fertilise.

If you do not have such a healthy pasture, you can 'take your horse out to eat' on verges, where a variety of plants can be found more and more often these days.

You can also pick plants and give them to your horse. Easy to find and good for your horse are nettle, thistle, common yarrow, cow parsley, cleavers, dandelion and ribwort plantain. Do not feed these plants in huge quantities. Some may contain a lot of fructan or more iron than is good for horses.

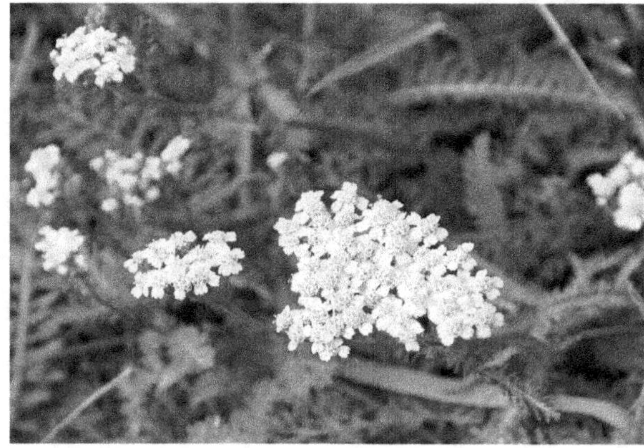

Common yarrow
(photo: Robert Dlesk)

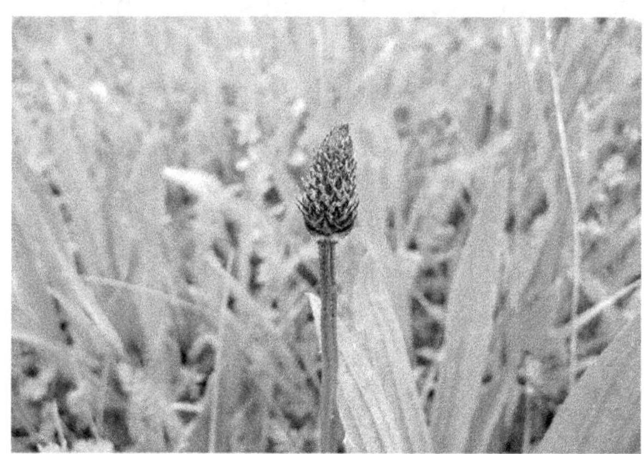

Ribwort plantain
(photo: Pavel Šinkyrík)

MICROBIOME

Accounting for 60%, the large intestine (colon) makes up the largest part of the horse's digestive system. Among other things, important vitamins are produced there. The colon is also the most important energy factory in the horse's body. Obviously, these processes should not be disturbed.

Disturbances in the gut microbiome are associated with reduced immunity, inflammation and laminitis. All of which you want to avoid at all costs in any horse – and especially one with PPID.

Factors that can knock the sensitive microbiome out of balance are sugar- and starch-rich diets with little fibre (grass full of sugar, cereals, pellets), feeding in meals, excessive exertion, diseases (especially colic), chronic worm infestation, medications (including antibiotics), worming treatments and residual fertilisers and pesticides.

Later in this chapter you will read about the importance of intelligent worming. With a PPID horse, do not stop worming for the sake of its intestinal health, but worm with policy.

Some people give probiotics ('good' bacteria) to improve bacterial balance in the gut. Commonly used are mannan-oligosaccharides, brewer's yeast and lactic acid bacilli. Scientific evidence that probiotics are effective is currently thin [138].

TREATMENT OF CLINICAL SIGNS AND COMPLICATIONS

On page 27 and beyond, you've read about all the clinical signs that plague the PPID horse. Some of these you will need to treat.

COAT MAINTENANCE, HYPER- AND HYPOHIDROSIS

To address both hypertrichosis and its effect on hyperhidrosis, many people shave or clip the coat of their PPID horse. Especially in the summer months or when the coat gets so long that it starts to molt, this can be much needed. Shaving may also help keep the skin healthy and detect and treat skin problems such as rain scab early. Regular brushing also helps to detect skin problems and wounds early.

Good clippers are pricey. It may be worth renting them or having someone come in who has the right equipment and experience.

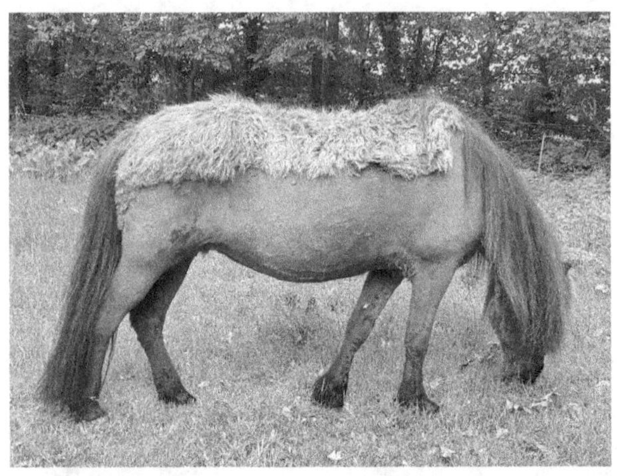

Pony with hypertrichosis, after a shave *(photo: Jacqueline Verhagen)*

Although healthy horses can almost always go through life without a blanket, for a shaved PPID horse in autumn and winter it is sometimes convenient or even necessary to wear a blanket to stay warm and dry. Sometimes a rain blanket or a medium-light turnout blanket (50 to 100 grams of fill) is enough. Just make sure your horse doesn't get too hot. This means you may have to put the blanket on and off several times a day.

Horses with severe hypertrichosis can regrow their coat very quickly. So again, be careful not to let them walk around with a blanket unnecessarily.

Besides PPID, aging horses experience diminished ability to regulate their body temperature. Consequently, they become less resilient to winter cold and more prone to discomfort in hot summer weather.

During summer, it's crucial to ensure that horses with hypertrichosis or hypohidrosis have access to shade at all times.

DENTAL CARE

The majority of PPID horses are of advanced age, and with aging comes certain flaws. Dental issues, including periodontitis, tooth loss, and abnormalities in wear such as hooks, are quite common. For older horses, dental care holds greater significance compared to their younger counterparts. In the context of PPID, this importance grows even further.

> PERIODONTITIS
> A category of inflammatory conditions affecting the supporting tissue of the teeth.

Simply pulling the tongue to one side to view the back molars is not a reliable and sometimes dangerous method of detecting dental abnormalities.

While many horses with PPID and EMS tend to be overweight, not all horses with PPID share this characteristic. Older horses often lean towards being underweight, and irregular dental care exacerbates their weight maintenance challenges.

In young, healthy horses, molars typically align well, forming a functional unit. Older horses commonly exhibit increased gaps between molars, known as diastemas. These spaces trap food, leading to issues like quidding and gum inflammation (gingivitis). Diastemas can also develop between front teeth, posing an immediate threat due to heightened susceptibility to inflammation. Consult your equine dentist for solutions to address this problem.

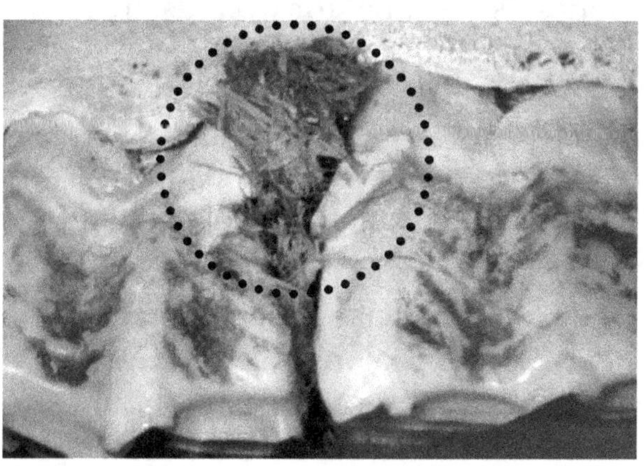

Quidding
(photo: Cedric Coucke)

On page 40 you have read about EOTRH. In horses suffering from this condition, regular dental check-ups and care by an equine dentist are very important. In certain instances, tooth extraction may be necessary.

Establishing a regular visit schedule with your equine dentist, customised to the specific requirements of a horse with PPID, is very good practice. A minimum of two visits per year is recommended.

INFECTION, INFLAMMATION AND WOUND CARE

Horses with PPID often have a weakened immune system, elevating the risk of infections. Swift and robust treatment, potentially involving antibiotics, is essential for wounds, infections, and inflammations.

Stay vigilant for the emergence of wounds, infections, and inflammations. A sinus infection (sinusitis), for instance, manifests with a foul smell and yellowish nasal discharge. Blankets and prolonged use of hoof boots can lead to rubbing and wounds. Weaker horses are sometimes harshly put in their place by herd mates. Bite and kick wounds are not rare.

Employing a fly mask, fly lamp, or other forms of fly control during summer can effectively minimise the risk of ocular infection.

If in doubt about the severity, always consult a vet for your horse. Timely intervention is very important, as a simple inflammation in a PPID horse can escalate rapidly.

SMEGMA

Build-up of smegma results in dirt in the sheath and on the inside of the hind legs. Regularly clean both areas with lukewarm water and a sponge. Additionally, remove the beans (refer to page 39). The horse should either have its penis naturally hanging out or you should gently pull it out. Use disposable gloves when cleaning the sheath. The accumulated smegma has quite a unpleasant smell.

Some geldings and stallions may not appreciate being touched in their private areas. With proper training, most can be accustomed to it. If needed, work together with someone who can lift a front leg while you clean, making it more difficult for the horse to kick with its hind leg.

Some horses may require mild sedation before any cleaning. If your horse is already sedated for dental maintenance, take advantage of the opportunity to perform the big clean.

WORMING

PPID-afflicted horses exhibit heightened vulnerability to worm infections. Wormicides have a shorter-lived effect on them compared to their healthy herdmates [132]. This susceptibility is linked to the diminished resistance associated with PPID.

Have regular faecal examinations done to determine the type and amount of parasites. A blood test to detect tapeworm is also advisable. Deworm diligently, following a schedule and with the right anthelmintics. Consult with your vet on how best to go about this.

VACCINATIONS

Ensure that vaccinations are up to date. PPID-affected horses may be more susceptible to infections, but they still have a good immune response to vaccination. Only for vaccines against rhino (rhinopneumonia/EHV) and West Nile virus this could be the case to a lesser extent [56].

LAMINITIS

If your horse is laminitic, take it off the pasture immediately. Put it in the paddock or riding arena and make sure it is comfortable and dry there. A thick layer of straw or sawdust will certainly please its feet.

Provide fresh drinking water. Give coarse-stemmed hay, preferably soaked in warm water (see sidebar on page 127). Do not give food high in sugar or starch; not even a handful of cereals or half an apple. Provide a salt lick. Optionally, give two tablespoons of iodine salt daily.

Supplement magnesium to increase insulin sensitivity [184]. If it turns out later that your horse is not insulin resistant, giving magnesium is not bad for the horse unless it has kidney problems.

First of all, call your vet and tell them that your horse has got both laminitis and PPID. Then call your hoof care provider to properly trim the hooves and, if necessary, take the shoes off first.

Consult with your hoof care provider about hoof boots. There are therapeutic hoof boots made especially for horses with laminitis. We will talk more about boots later. If you do not have hoof boots yet, you can make emergency hoof pads to bridge the gap. There is a simple guide in the sidebar on the next page. Your hoof care provider will undoubtedly be willing to do this for you, if you are not so handy yourself.

The severity of your horse's condition will determine whether the vet recommends treatment in the clinic. Horses severely affected by laminitis, unable to stand for extended periods or even get up at all are better off in the clinic than at home. This is especially true if there are serious complications, such as a sole perforation or hoof sloughing (the detachment of the entire hoof capsule). A horse with such problems needs more comprehensive care and monitoring than you can manage at home.

EMERGENCY HOOF PADS

A gardening kneeling pad can quickly be transformed into emergency hoof pads
to temporarily protect your horse's painful hooves:

- Make sure the hoof is clean, dry and preferably correctly trimmed.
- Place the hoof on the kneeling pad.
- Use a marker to trace the outline of the hoof on the pad.
- Cut it out.
- Lift the hoof and place the cut-out pad under it. Use duct tape to attach. First use a strip of tape going from one side of the hoof the other side, keeping the hoof pad in place.
- Lay a gauze on the heel bulbs to protect them from the glue from the duct tape. Now wrap the hoof and pad with tape. Be careful not to tape the coronary band.

Stable rest is seldom an ideal solution. In the stable, your horse may not move adequately, leading to insufficient hoof perfusion. Then there is stress, triggering unwanted hormonal effects, including an increase in ACTH and cortisol. Stabling, particularly for horses accustomed to outdoor living, can be a source of stress.

Ensure your horse can move carefully and according to its needs. However, avoid this if your horse is in such poor condition that any movement induces pain. Consult with your vet to determine appropriate pain relief strategies.

If you do not have a paddock or riding arena at your disposal to put your horse in, a temporary solution can sometimes be made with electric tape in the yard. Perhaps you can pull a few stalls together to create a loose stable for your horse.

Of course, there are also situations where stable rest is more important for recovery than exercise. Take serious complications, such as a sole perforation, for example. Engage in discussions with your vet to determine how to minimise stall rest in such scenarios.

HOOF CARE FOR THE LAMINITIC HORSE
Although laminitis is probably not a direct clinical manifestation of PPID, but a consequence of EMS/insulin dysregulation, we consider it as such in this book. Assuming the most positive statistics, one in three PPID horses also has EMS/ID, posing a significant risk of endocrinopathic laminitis.

During its initial stages, endocrinopathic laminitis tends to be less painful than the other two forms (SIRS-related and traumatic). However, without intervention, it will progressively become intensely painful and result in significant damage to the hooves. Regular and expert hoof care is vital for a horse with laminitis. Hoof care includes trimming, hoof protection and treatment of the complications of laminitis.

TRIMMING

Trimming a laminitic hoof is hardly any different from trimming a healthy one. In both cases, a modern hoof care provider focuses on balancing the hoof, improving its shape and optimising the distribution of forces. In the case of laminitis, this reduces pain, improves the hoof mechanism and thus leads to faster recovery. Simply put, the goal of trimming is to grow a healthy hoof capsule around the internal foot. Consider the hoof capsule as the shoe of the internal foot. The better this shoe fits, the better your horse moves, the faster it heals.

If necessary, flip back to page 47 to refresh your knowledge of equine hoof anatomy.

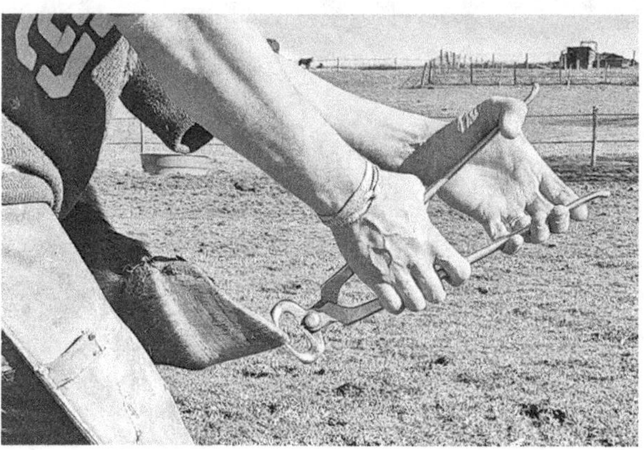

Because the back of the hoof is generally unaffected by laminitis, we want the horse to bear its weight there. This provides good shock absorption, good circulation and ensures that the hoof properly breaks over.
A second and very important goal of trimming is to take the pressure off the damaged lamellar connection so that it can grow back into a healthy state.

We also do not want pressure from the coffin bone from the inside on the sole. The latter two points require the coffin bone to be parallel to the ground when the horse loads its hoof in motion.

We cannot, of course, explain in one small page how all this is done, but in general it comes down to this:

- The heels are kept low, positioned in line with the widest part of the frog as quickly as possible, and possibly slightly bevelled. Your hoof care provider tries to promote heel first landing this way. Also, the coffin bone will come parallel to the ground in this way
- The pressure in the quarters (sides) of the hoof is taken off to improve the health of the hoof cartilages (collateral cartilages)
- The hoof wall in the toe area is trimmed and rounded off to keep it off the ground and to minimise stress on the damaged lamellar connection. If necessary, the lamellar wedge (see sidebar on page 69) is partially rasped away.

- Flares are removed as they generate excessive stress to the lamellar connection as well.
- Normal sole tissue remains untouched because all healthy sole provides valuable cushioning
- The bars are trimmed to reduce pressure on sensitive tissues in the hoof.
- The frog retains its function as a shock absorber and carries a considerable part of the weight. Where it blocks the collateral grooves, your hoof care provider will trim it back. Dirt must be able to get out of the grooves.
- Parts of the frog and white line that are affected by bacteria or fungi are cut clean and treated.

FREQUENCY

Laminitic hooves need to be trimmed much more frequently than those of a healthy horse. In the beginning, your hoof care provider will be on your doorstep every three weeks. Later, that may be cut down to every five weeks.

In between visits, you may need to pick up a hoof rasp to do some maintenance yourself (see sidebar on the next page). Your hoof care provider will explain to you exactly what to do and what not to do.

As long as the shape and balance of the hoof are not restored, the force acting on the damaged tissues in the hoof will perpetuate the problem.

Your hoof care provider will want to remedy this as quickly as possible. That is why they suggest visiting so often.

The remedy should not be worse than the disease. Lowering high heels, for example, is not something to be done in one go, but rather in stages. That way too much tension on the deep flexor tendon can be prevented. Also, the hoof can be so deformed that the blood flow is pinched off. Certain amino acids that are important for hoof growth do not get to the right places in the hoof at the same time. This causes your horse to have cup-shaped hooves with high heels. Frequent trimming helps to solve this problem.

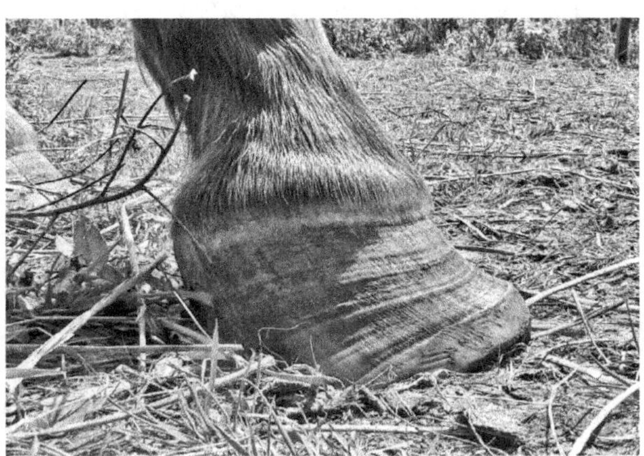

Cup-shaped hoof with high heels

WHAT CAN I DO MYSELF BETWEEN TRIMMING APPOINTMENTS?

Trimming a laminitic hoof requires experience, insight, knowledge and skill that very few horse owners have. Essentially because it is generally the first time that they may have had to deal with such a hoof. Preferably this is why you should leave it to a professional hoof care provider, even if you trim your other horses' hooves yourself. In close consultation with your hoof care provider however, you can still do useful work in between their visits. They can explain how to keep the toes of the hoof short so that they do not touch the ground. That way, there is no pressure on the damaged lamellar connection, which speeds up the healing process. The same applies to flares.

Complications such as thrush or white line disease should be treated daily. You can do that after your hoof care provider has cut the area clean and started the treatment. They will tell you which products to use.

Never try to cut or rasp a laminitic hoof on your own. There is the potential that inadvertently you will do more harm than good before you know it. Ask your hoof care provider if there is anything you can do and, more importantly, how you can do it. Be prepared to let them also judge your work.

There are plentiful courses readily available these days that teach you the basics of trimming. It is a good idea to take such a course before attempting to work on your horses. For the sake of completeness, we would like to state explicitly that such a course does not train you to become a professional hoof care provider. It only serves to equip you even better for hoof care between visits from your farrier.

It is expensive to have your hoof care provider come so often, but you get what you pay for. Skimping on hoof care will slow down the healing process considerably. In the end, you might end up with vet bills that are much higher than those of your hoof care provider.

HOOF PROTECTION

Hoof protection includes the temporary or long-term application of materials or objects to or around the hoof to provide comfort, reduce wear, alter force distribution and, in the case of laminitis, accelerate healing or at least halt the progression of the condition.

HOOF BOOTS

Using hoof boots is a way to get through the period of healing properly, quickly and pain-free. It's a temporary aid that becomes redundant over time. If your PPID-afflicted horse, then hoof boots should really come into the picture immediately. Why subject your horse to unnecessary pain when it can be easily alleviated?

IS A HOOF CARE PROVIDER SOMETHING ELSE THAN A FARRIER?

Trimmer, farrier, and even equine podiatrist; these are all names for professionals dedicated to horse hoof care, and they are all colleagues too.

As soon as someone, in a professional setting, touches a horse's feet with a pair of nippers, a rasp and a hoof knife, he or she is a hoof care provider. So, this is the broadest term.

If it involves shoeing, then you are dealing with a farrier. The shoes can be made of iron or synthetic materials, and the farrier can try to imitate bare feet with them. Hoof boots are considered part of the barefoot approach. After use, they can be removed and stored. Glue-on synthetic shoes and boots are something in between. Both trimmers and farriers use them.

Pain-free exercise enhances blood flow to all tissues in the hoof. Proper movement expedites the disappearance of fluid accumulation (oedema) in the affected hoof tissue. The recovery of an inflamed and hypersensitive sole dermis is accelerated with the use of boots. Horses equipped with boots experience fewer hoof abscesses. Additionally, it's important to note that exercise aids in burning sugars, contributing to weight loss. Furthermore, exercise enhances sensitivity to insulin [85].

With boots, the hoof undergoes alternating pressure and pressure relief, which is known as the hoof mechanism. This alternation occurs between the moment the hoof bears the horse's weight and the moment the hoof is free from the ground. This mechanism is a key element in blood circulation in the hoof and the horse's leg. In therapeutic metal hoof shoes with frog support, such as heartbar shoes, this particular element of hoof mechanism is virtually non-existent as the frog is under constant pressure.

Boots enable a quicker return to doing fun, active things with your horse. For some horses, breaking the cycle of laminitis, healing, and recurrence is achievable with the use of boots. It won't be the first time a horse escapes euthanasia thanks to boots.

Another great thing about boots is that they can be taken off after use. This allows regular hoof trimming at short intervals. This contrasts with therapeutic shoes, which, as time passes since the farrier's visit, lose the intended effect as they grow away from the problem as it were.

The hoof care provider or boot fitter can apply all kinds of insoles for optimal protection and shock absorption for your horse's painful hooves.

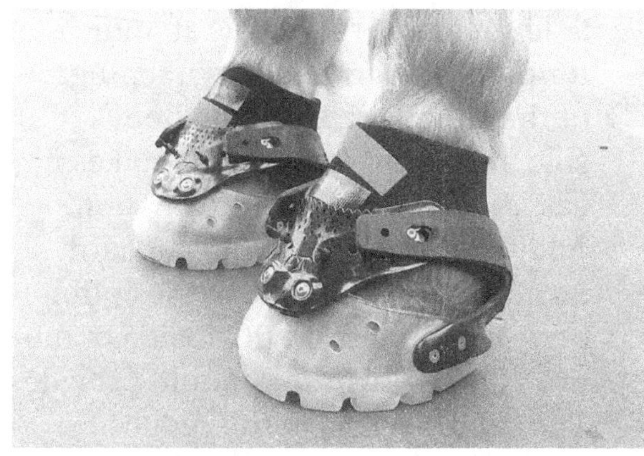

Hoof boots for riding
(photo: Mirjam van Hoorn)

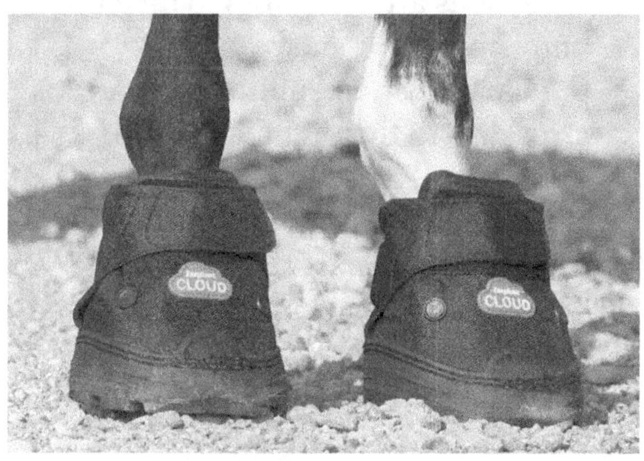

Therapeutic hoof boots
(photo: Valley Vet Supply)

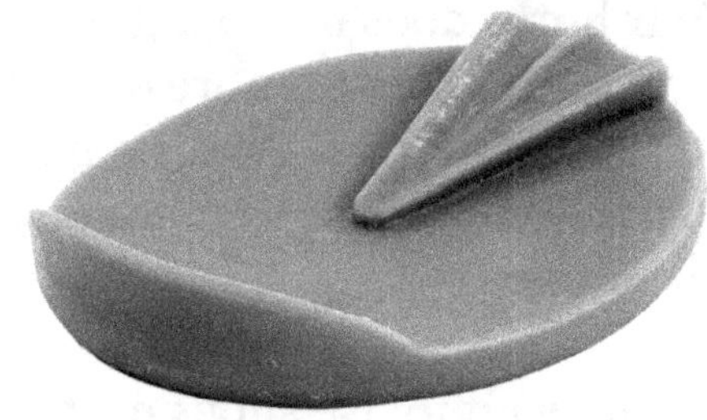

Insole with frog support
(photo: Soft-ride)

Additionally, it's possible to cut and rasp the sole of the boot to precisely position the break-over point.

With the exception of therapeutic models, hoof boots aren't designed for continuous wear. If you want to attempt this anyway, opt for lightweight shoes that fit perfectly without causing any rubbing. Water should drain easily. Protect the coronary band and hoof bulbs, if needed, using a self-adhesive bandage, socks, or a small amount of Vaseline.

Modern hoof protection exists that combines features of boots and synthetic glue-on shoes. Essentially, it's like a glued-on boot. While the downside is the lack of possibility to regularly trim the hooves, the upside is the continuous 24/7 protection they provide.

THERAPEUTIC SHOEING

In farriery, therapeutic shoes are commonly used for laminitis cases, primarily aiming for symptomatic relief. While certain therapeutic shoes may positively impact specific anatomical aspects or biomechanical functions of hoof tissues, it doesn't eliminate all the disadvantages associated with shoeing. In fact, there are numerous drawbacks to using hoof shoes.

DISADVANTAGES

The hoof mechanism cannot function optimally, whereas this is so important for the healing of laminitis. A second major problem is that all the force that the hoof exerts on the ground is transmitted via the shoe to the lamellar connection. This is precisely the damaged tissue that is unable to absorb this force. This is what we call peripheral loading.

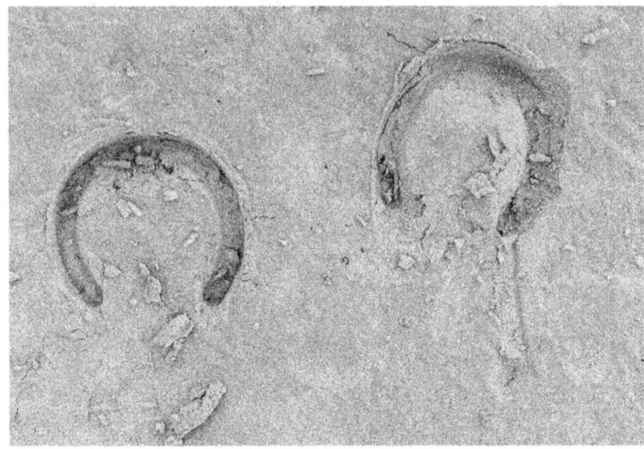

Peripheral loading due to shoeing

We will now pick from the list of other disadvantages of shoes:
- Between shoeing appointments, the hoof wall cannot be trimmed. As a result, it can rapidly lengthen, causing it to pull on the lamellar connection like a lever.
- The horseshoe is nailed, screwed or glued to the partially loose hoof wall. This is in the process of healing to regrow healthy tissue. The stress from the shoe hampers the growth of the healthy tissue, specifically the lamellar connection, causing it to 'tear' loose.

- Sole sensitivity serves as an indicator of improvement or worsening of the situation. The shod hoof's sole, being off the ground, makes it easy to overlook this information. Additionally, the sole fails to harden adequately, depriving the coffin bone pressing from the inside of the protection a firm sole would provide.
- The same applies to the reduced flexibility of the sole in a shod hoof. The risk of sole bruises and hoof abscesses increases. This makes the horse even more sensitive than it already is and less able to take the movement it needs.
- A heartbar shoe applies constant pressure to the digital cushion, whereas this tissue requires a balance of alternating pressure and relief for optimal health.
- Shoes with raised branches or wedges aimed at easing tension in the deep flexor tendon actually heighten pressure on the tip of the hoof bone. This results in increased force on the damaged lamellar connection in the toe region of the hoof.
- There is less sensation in the hooves. Your horse does not feel the ground it walks on. It trips more often and occasionally slips. This is painful, so it will move less than is good for him.

If you still want to use shoes despite all the disadvantages mentioned above, choose plastic over metal and glue rather than nails.

To be honest, the temptation to shoe a laminitic horse is understandable. After all, the horse suddenly seems to be able to walk reasonably pain-free. However, this makes it walk more, longer and faster than the recovering tissues can handle. The apparent short-term gain of relief in pain is overshadowed by slower long-term healing.

SYNTHETIC SHOES

There are both hoof care providers and farriers who offer synthetic shoes. This type of hoof protection can be all plastic or have a metal core. The former variant is then better than the latter. If it is glued, it is better than if it is nailed.

As with metal shoes, there are therapeutic variants with frog support and open toe shoes.

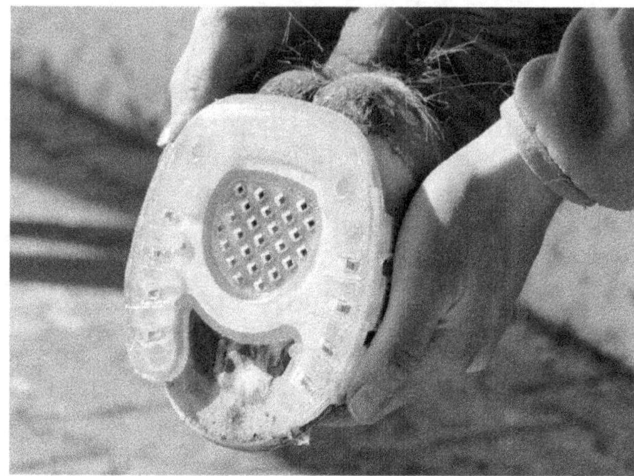

Synthetic therapeutic shoes
(photo: Duplo)

Synthetic shoes share some disadvantages with traditional metal ones. Some of these downsides also apply to hoof boots, by the way. One is the inertial force (which is also what one feels when sitting in a car that suddenly turns sharply) that acts on bones, joints and small blood vessels. To which we should add that in the recovery period of laminitis, the horse is likely to move only in stride. That inertia force will not be so bad.

Just like with regular shoes, peripheral loading occurs. With synthetic shoes, your horse will not feel the ground properly either and may therefore trip more often. Regular trimming of the hooves to keep the toes short and the heels low is not feasible too. Shoes, no matter what material, increase the toe length and therefore the leverage on the painful lamellar connection.

COMPLICATIONS OF LAMINITIS

Laminitis comes with its own specific complications that require care and attention.

ABSCESSES

Cutting open a hoof abscess and draining pus gives immediate relief. It is essential that this treatment is conducted under sterile conditions, making it a task for the veterinarian rather than the hoof care provider. The latter does not have sterile tools and they cannot provide the aftercare that is needed. If mishandled, there's a risk of new abscesses, infection, or even sepsis.

The vet first determines where the abscess is located and how thick the surrounding tissues (sole, white line, hoof wall) are through hoof testers or X-ray. Following this, they create one or several small openings to drain pus from the abscess, followed by a thorough rinsing with disinfectant.

Post abscess incision, meticulous cleaning of the hoof with iodine, for instance, is imperative. This daily cleaning routine should continue for at least a week, or as long as required to ensure the wound is entirely clean. Additionally, the vet will inquire about your horse's tetanus shot status.

Alternatively, one can wait for the abscess to mature and rupture naturally, avoiding the need for incision. To make this happen faster, some people soak the hoof in warm water with green soap. While this is effective, keep in mind that it weakens the sole and white line, elevating the risk of new bacterial entry and potential development of a septic abscess.

An abscess may find its way out through the coronary band. The hole that this will create will then grow downwards with the hoof wall.

Keep an eye on that spot. It is possible that a fungus will settle in it. If so, treatment with a fungicide is necessary. Often, white kitchen vinegar with a few drops of tea tree oil will do the trick.

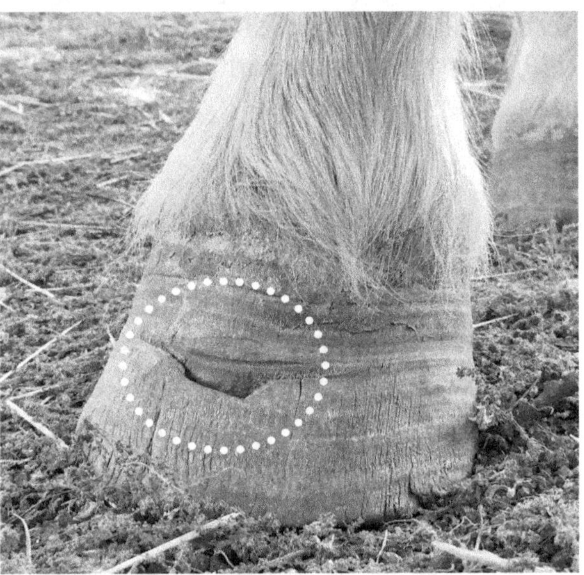

Old abscess outbreak

OSTEITIS

Unfortunately, advanced laminitis often leads to severe complications. Addressing them falls under the purview of the veterinarian or veterinary surgeon. Osteitis is one such complication. It is an inflammation of the bone. In particular, osteitis of the coffin bone is a common complication in advanced chronic laminitis.

In septic osteitis (where germs are present), surgical curettage and flushing of the bone are necessary. With the aseptic variant, this is not the case.

SOLE PERFORATION

The coffin bone can rotate, sink and press on the sole from the inside to such an extent that the sole is no longer able to withstand this pressure. In such cases, the tip of the bone penetrates the sole, becoming visible externally; a condition known as sole perforation. This is a painful complication with a heightened risk of infection.

Your hoof care provider, in consultation or cooperation with the veterinarian, will strive to optimise the position of the coffin bone to prevent worsening of the situation. The wound will be properly cleaned and the hoof appropriately bandaged. Hoof boots may be employed, and in areas where the exposed coffin bone contacts the boot, a notch can be cut in the sole of the latter. The boot must be kept clean and disinfected well at all times. The veterinarian prescribes antibiotics for the horse.

WHITE LINE DISEASE

This condition involves an infection of the hoof wall and sometimes the underlying tissues, caused by a combination of bacteria and fungi. Your hoof care provider is equipped to address this issue. Often, the affected part of the hoof wall is removed. After that, this spot needs to be treated regularly by you. There are all kinds of products available for this, both old tried-and-tested household remedies

and professional products. Depending on how severe the infestation is, your hoof care provider or vet will decide which approach is best. Avoid just picking a remedy yourself, as more potent solutions increase the risk of drying out and affecting healthy or regenerating tissues.

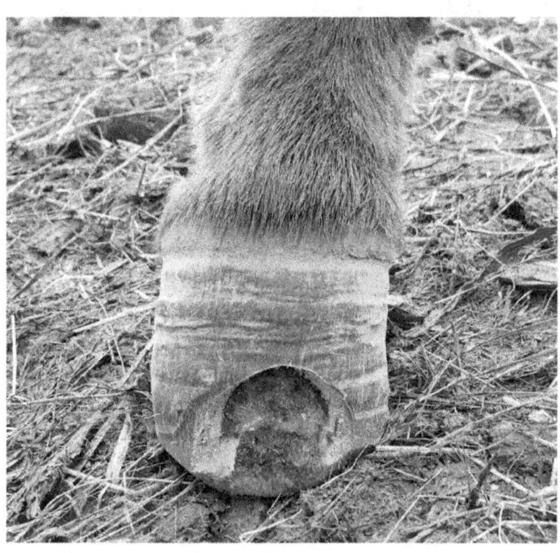

Severe white line disease in a donkey

It is good to understand that white line disease can only manifest when the hoof wall's horn is already of poor quality. Bacteria and fungi are not the primary causes. Try to find out why the quality of the horn tissue is subpar. Deficiencies in specific trace elements and amino acids, and an imbalanced ratio of iron, copper, zinc, and manganese, are correlated with poor horn tissue.

Mechanical causes, like an excessively long hoof wall or stance abnormalities overloading the hoof wall, can induce damage, creating opportunities for fungal access. A deformed hoof wall, as seen in laminitis cases, is also a recognised cause.

Substances in the horse's manure and urine deteriorate the horn cells. Excessively wet ground or bedding makes the sole and white line too soft, while too dry hooves are prone to tearing. The fungus directly thrives in such conditions. Old nail holes are also often the starting point of white line disease.

SURGICAL TREATMENT

When the vet starts talking about surgical intervention to control chronic laminitis, you can be sure the condition is in advanced stages. A tenotomy and hoof wall resection are the most commonly used surgical procedures.

TENOTOMY

In a tenotomy procedure, the veterinary surgeon severs the deep flexor tendon. The aim is to remove the tractive force exerted by the tendon on the coffin bone, thereby addressing coffin bone rotation. It should be noted here that the tension of the deep flexor tendon is not the primary cause of the rotation. The main issue lies in the inability of the lamellar connection, along with the extensor tendon, to counteract the downward pressure of the horse's body weight.

Potential complications, including swelling, pain, bone inflammation, connective tissue proliferation (overgrowth), osteoarthritis, joint deformities, and permanent tendon contraction, may arise. Extensive and prolonged aftercare is necessary.

HOOF WALL RESECTION

Resection entails the removal of a portion of the hoof wall, a procedure carried out by the farrier at the veterinary clinic to alleviate pressure and enhance blood circulation, ultimately promoting better hoof growth.

However, this should only be considered if the vet or farrier deems it absolutely necessary. The procedure carries risks such as inflammation, abscesses, or tissue overgrowth. Moreover, it can lead to excessive pressure on the remaining hoof wall. If the entire lamellar connection is compromised, opting for resection might only prolong the issue, increasing the likelihood of coffin bone rotation or sinking.

MOVEMENT AND EXERCISE

What we said earlier about nutrition also applies to exercise. It is one of the aspects of your horse's living conditions that you can have complete control over. A significant benefit is that, as a treatment approach, it comes at no expense.

HOW DO I KNOW WHEN LAMINITIS IS OVER?

The first indication that (the acute phase of) laminitis might be over is when you no longer see the clinical signs described on page 69 (sidebar 'Recognising laminitis'). Obel 0 (see page 71) is also good news, of course. Your hoof care provider is trained to notice things that you might overlook. If you have any doubts, consult with them to see if they think the worst is over.

If you really want to be sure, your veterinarian can perform a clinical examination again. Blood test results and X-rays are very enlightening too. The latter in particular show when chronic laminitis is no longer present. Your vet can also tell you whether your horse really is no longer laminitic or whether it is only the clinical signs that have been successfully suppressed. The amount of pain, for example, is not the best indicator of the horse's condition. Some horses will not show signs of pain even when there is still tissue damage.

Aging horses tend to be less active than their younger counterparts. Not least because they are ridden less often. For them, but certainly also for younger horses affected by PPID, exercise is important for health in general and for muscles, tendons and hooves in particular.

Only exercise if your horse is physically capable, with well-trimmed hooves and, if needed, hoof boots equipped with soft insoles. Exercise should be approached cautiously, especially in horses with laminitis or those recently recovering from it. With them, you should be extra careful or even delaying exercise for a period. The laminitis has weakened the hoof and it takes a while for the body to fix that. Be patient and allow the hoof to stabilise before reintroducing your horse to work (see sidebar above).

The surface you let your horse move on should also be comfortable. Moving with sore feet on a bumpy, hard frozen meadow is an extreme example of is an extreme example of what to avoid.

Facilitate exercise through activities such as walking your horse, engaging in ground work, playing, or working under saddle. Adjust the intensity and duration of the latter based on what your horse is able to do. Introduce changes to the exercise and training program gradually.

Even without you present, you can provide more exercise. Foster social interaction with other horses, strategically place hay feeders, drinking water, and salt licks far apart, create a path in the pasture or arena using electric tape, or establish a paddock paradise (see sidebar on the next page).

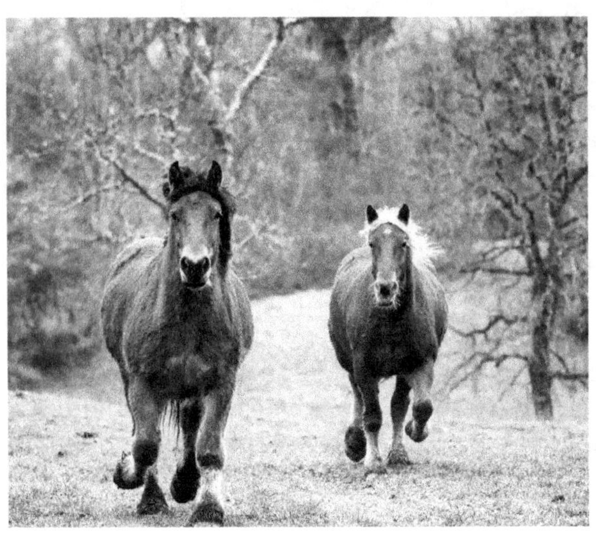

Moving more when together
(photo: Mandy Fontana)

EMS/INSULIN DYSREGULATION

Exercise holds particular significance for horses dealing with both PPID and EMS/insulin dysregulation, regardless of their weight status. While some studies indicate that increased exercise may not consistently result in long-term elevated insulin sensitivity [72], others suggest the opposite [67, 85, 128, 148, 154].

The latter are in the majority and mostly more recent. They support the conclusion that exercise contributes to enhanced insulin sensitivity, even in the absence of weight loss.

PADDOCK PARADISE

A paddock paradise is an environment that provides as much as is possible of the natural social, nutritional and exercise needs of a horse. The idea is based on the fact that in the wild, horses always follow the same fixed routes that connect watering holes, grazing areas, minerals and other interesting elements.

The starting point is a wide track around the field, connected here and there to a number of larger paddocks or pieces of pasture. Along the route, you can create all kinds of natural elements and challenges to stimulate movement. For example, you can place slow feeders, water troughs and salt licks far apart from each other and build walk-in stables or natural shelters. You can integrate hedgerows or tree lines.

Different kinds of surfaces with pavers, concrete slabs, pea gravel and rocks are also common in the paddock paradise. Although, for a horse with sensitive hooves, this may not always be the best choice, as it can cause overloading and pain. If these are already present in your paddock paradise, you can replace them with rubber mats or fence them off with a safe fence.

One last thing: it is highly unlikely that your horse will get the exercise it needs just by trudging through a paddock paradise, particularly if it needs to lose weight. Additional work will need to be undertaken.

Adiponectin increases with exercise. This improves insulin sensitivity. Exercise also lowers leptin concentrations in the blood. The benefits of this are explained on page 44.

The benefits of this are explained on page 44.

Hormonal improvements do not magically persist if the exercise programme is not continued.

For overweight horses, of course, exercise also simply results in weight loss.

Thirty minutes of exercise a day, five days a week, at moderate intensity, is recommended. By moderate intensity, we mean fast trot and gallop, whether under saddle or not.

Even low-intensity exercise can have positive effects, according to recent research [154]. A 2014 study saw an improvement in terms of inflammatory activity in horses trotting for five minutes a day for 14 days [67]. Of course, this does not mean that a low-intensity exercise programme is sufficient as a standard for all overweight horses. By low intensity we mean walk and trot, not under saddle. The overlap between low and moderate intensity lies partly in the speed of the trot.

In horses recently recovered from laminitis, low-intensity exercise on soft ground for about 30 minutes, three times a week is the norm. Again: only if your horse can handle it, on properly trimmed hooves and preferably on hoof boots with soft insoles.

COMPLEMENTARY THERAPIES

Besides all the treatment options described so far, there is a host of complementary or alternative therapies available to restore hormonal balance, optimise sugar metabolism, reduce pain, reduce inflammation or 'balance the whole body'. It is absolutely beyond the scope of this book to review or assess all these options for their therapeutic value or their scientific basis. If you feel comfortable with these forms of treatment, you might consider applying them in treating the clinical signs of PPID. Just be careful that they do not interfere with the treatment described in this book.

Be cautious of assertions about the effectiveness of any treatment solely based on improvements in clinical signs. Clinical improvement would probably also already occur merely by improving living conditions and overall health.

Complementary therapies are often endorsed citing scientific studies that lack an accurate diagnosis of PPID in the horses studied. The research design also leaves something to be desired a little too often. But let's be candid; quite a few studies investigating conventional remedies and therapies are also prone to these shortcomings.

A good example of all three of these points is an oft-cited study on the efficacy of homoeopathy [44]. The reported success rate in the horses involved was 91%. Unfortunately, the study solely focused on improvement in the clinical picture. Additionally, horses included in the study were diagnosed with PPID based solely on their blood sugar levels (!) and the clinical manifestation of hypertrichosis. It seems plausible that the dogs had Cushing's disease, not PPID, illustrating a classic case of comparing apples with oranges.

While ACTH was measured in some dogs to determine their eligibility, it was not done uniformly for all. Whether the remedy was effective was then not determined with a second measurement. In the horses, ACTH levels were neither measured before nor after the study in the horses, which would be expected, especially with treatment involving a product named 'ACTH 30c'. Lastly, there was no control group in this study.

AVOIDING STRESS

Elevated stress levels result in increased cortisol production, which, in turn, suppresses immune responses. Horses with PPID already have compromised immune systems. Cortisol further converts proteins and fats into sugar (glucose) and is linked to the development and exacerbation of insulin resistance. This is particularly detrimental for horses dealing with both PPID and ID. On page 52, you've learned that cortisol damages the hemidesmosomes of the basement membrane, contributing to the onset and development of laminitis.

Stress additionally elevates ACTH production in the anterior lobe of the pituitary gland. Adrenaline production also increases.

Hyperlipidaemia is also linked to chronic stress, as is decrease in antioxidant enzyme activity and hence increase in oxidative stress.

STRESS FACTORS

Possible stressors you could address are:
- Pain, including that arising from the clinical signs of PPID in general and specifically from laminitis and its complications
- Transportation
- Competition
- Chronic worm infestation
- Veterinarian consultation, rushed or grumpy farrier, dentist

- Poorly fitting saddle
- Monotonous or excessive training, with regular training for a horse experiencing muscle atrophy due to PPID considered as excessive
- A stressful bond with the rider or trainer
- Lack of balanced social interaction: no herd or alone in box, or too many changes in the herd
- A stressful relationship with another herdmate, hierarchy problems, being rejected from the herd
- Restless living environment. For example, a busy livery yard or a pasture next to a motorway.
- Mourning. Two horses that have grown up together or that have chosen each other as buddy who are suddenly separated
- Age. Older horses seem less able to cope with stressful situations

EUTHANASIA

No horse has ever died of PPID itself. The ethical dilemma arises from the severity and prolonged nature of complications, coupled with the progressive aspect of PPID, leaving little room for improvement. This prompts reflection on whether it is ethical to continue sustaining the horse's life. Your horse cannot tell you itself when it has had enough.

While the final decision rests with you, the veterinarian is in the best position to provide objective assessments of your horse's current and future well-being. They can offer a broader perspective by comparing your horse's situation with others they have encountered in their practice.

The vet will make an objective assessment, looking at the nature and severity of complications again. They will critically assess the chosen treatment methods and their efficacy, particularly focusing on pain management in severe laminitis cases. They will consult with your horse's other practitioners such as the hoof care provider and the dentist. They will be honest enough to also consider the extent to which you are able to provide the necessary care. If, for whatever reason, it is not possible to help your horse properly, then it is not fair to let it suffer. It is up to you to decide what the outcome will be in that case.

It is a difficult decision to make, one that often takes more time with the owner than what the veterinarian considers desirable from the horse's interest. Fortunately, veterinarians understand that this is part of their job. They will afford you the necessary time to reflect on their advice.

During this process, you should not hesitate to ask them again, if necessary, to substantiate this advice, or request the opinion of another veterinarian.

If you really cannot yet part with your horse, terminal care may still be an option. However, whether this approach would genuinely benefit your horse is another matter.

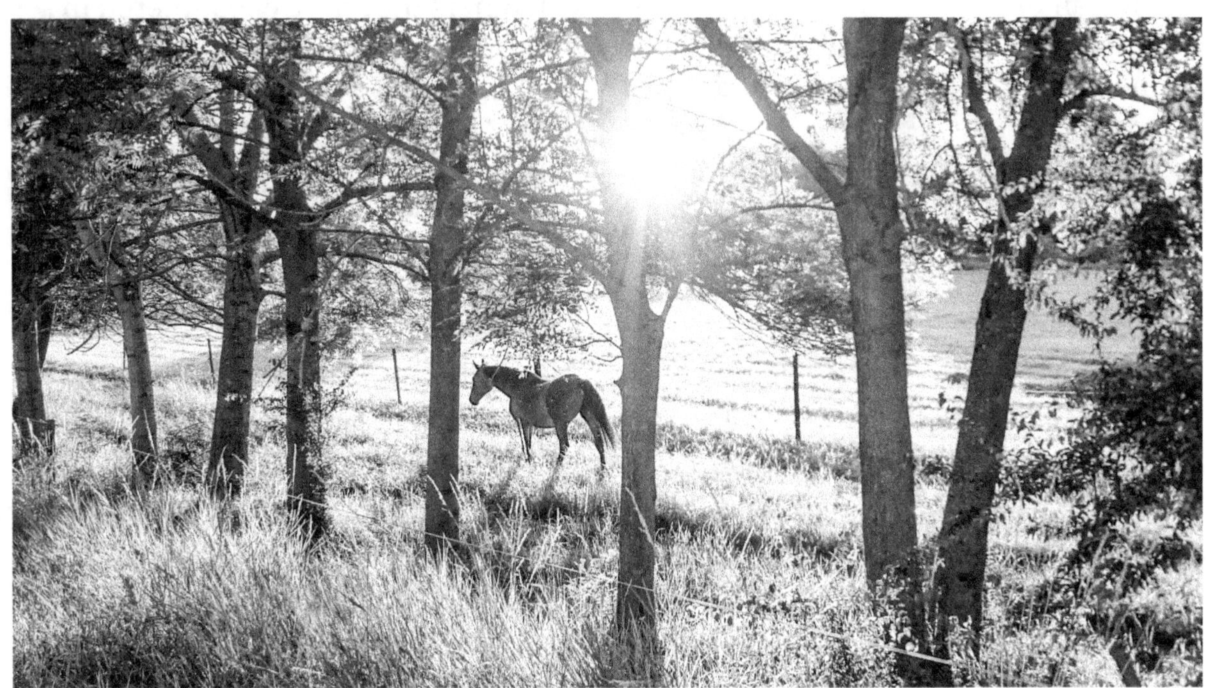

(photo: Flash Dantz)

SUMMARY

Treatment of PPID includes the use of drugs as well as attention to general healthcare and adjustments in living conditions. By general healthcare, we mean deworming and vaccination, among other things. Hoof care, dental care and treatment of any other complications is also very important. Weight control is part of the management of EMS and laminitis.

The lack of dopamine can be supplemented synthetically with the dopamine agonist pergolide. This is well tolerated by most horses, but not all. In some horses, the side effects are worse than the disease. Chasteberry is an herbal remedy that can suppress certain clinical signs. It does not lower ACTH levels.

For the complications of PPID, the veterinarian can also employ a variety of medications. Plant-based alternatives exist for many drugs. Scientific evidence for their efficacy is still scarce. The same applies to the use of antioxidants.

Nutrition and exercise are important weapons in the fight against EMS, weight problems and muscle breakdown. Ageing and dental problems call for different food or feeding methods. In fact, no PPID-affected equine escapes a modified diet.

At the end of the journey, for many horses with PPID, euthanasia is the very last thing you can do for them.

CLEOPATRA

The stunning mare on the cover of this book is Cleopatra. A horse that, despite her PPID, radiates strength and hope. It is my personal hope that this image can serve to encourage the readers of my book and give them the extra incentive not to give up too quickly.

Cleopatra has reached the respectable age of 37 years. Photographer Nikkie de Kerf has captured Cleopatra so beautifully.

ACKNOWLEDGEMENTS

Equine nutritionist Suzanne Buijsse has contributed enormously to everything about nutrition, PPID and laminitis in this book; she really made me think differently about several things. In addition she also helped me to keep me in line when I threatened to get too technical.

Veterinarian Gaelle Selfslagh helped ensure that the 'Description' and 'Causes' chapters were correct.

Heleen Davies was the right person to point out the blind spots I had developed in my own field of horse feet.

Equine dentist Cedric Coucke cut his teeth on the text on dental problems, providing huge clarity in that section.

Many thanks to Monika Danielak for her meticulous language corrections, which have greatly enhanced this book.

I am also extremely grateful to all the photographers for the beautiful and unique photos I was permitted to include to illustrate the chapters of this book.

Thank you all so much! Thanks to you I can make such fine books.

Clermont-Ferrand, July 2024

Remco Sikkel

RESOURCES

BOOKS

Clinical equine oncology / C. Knottenbelt. – 2015, ISBN : 978-0-7020-4266-9
Current therapy in equine medicine / E. Robinson. – 2015, ISBN : 1-4557-4555-3
Diagnostic techniques in equine medicine / G. Frank. – 2009, ISBN : 978-0-7020-2792-5
Equine applied and clinical nutrition / R. Geor. – 2013, ISBN : 978-0-7020-3422-0
Equine laminitis / J. Belknap. – 2017, ISBN : 978-1-119-16909-3
Hoefbevangenheid : begrijpen, genezen, voorkomen / R. Sikkel. – 2018, ISBN : 978-90-825191-9-8
The horse nutrition handbook / M. Worth. - 2010, ISBN : 1-60342-541-1
PPID and your horse : an owner information guide / Boehringer-Ingelheim. – 2019
PPID : ja of nee / A. Wiertz, J. Driessen. – 2020, ISBN : 1-230-00440-8
Saunders handbook of veterinary drugs : small and large animal / M. Papich. – 2015, ISBN : 0-323-24485-8

ARTICLES

1. 3-Nitrotyrosine: a versatile oxidative stress biomarker for major neurodegenerative diseases / M. Bandookwala, P. Sengupta, *Int J Neurosci* 130 (2020): 1047–1062

2. 4 Hydroxyisoleucine : a plant-derived treatment for metabolic syndrome / L. Jetté, L. Harvey, K. Eugeni (et al.), *Curr Opin Investig Drugs* 10 (2009): 353–358

3. The accuracy of ACTH as a biomarker for pituitary pars intermedia dysfunction in horses : a systematic review and meta-analysis / J. Meyer, L. Hunyadi, J. Ordóñez-Mena, *Equine Vet J* (2021)

4. Adipokine, chemokine, and cytokine expression profiles in adipose tissue depots of lean and overweight ponies / P. Weber, K. Schermerhorn, L. McCutcheon (et al.), *J Equine Vet Sci* 33 (2013): 846

5. Adrenocorticotropin concentration following administration of thyrotropin-releasing hormone in healthy horses and those with pituitary pars intermedia dysfunction and pituitary gland hyperplasia / J. Beech, R. Boston, S. Lindborg (et al.), *J Am Vet Med Assoc* 231 (2007): 417–426

6. Advantages and limitations of the equine disease, pituitary pars intermedia dysfunction as a model of spontaneous dopaminergic neurodegenerative disease / D. McFarlane, *Ageing Res Rev* 6 (2007): 54–63

7. Aging effect on plasma metabolites and hormones concentrations in riding horses / K. Kawasumi, M. Yamamoto, M. Koide (et al.), *Open Vet J* 5 (2015): 154–157

8. Agnus castus extracts inhibit prolactin secretion of rat pituitary cells / G. Sliutz, P. Speiser, A. Schultz (et al.), *Horm Metab Res* 25 (1993): 253–255

9. Alpha-melanocyte stimulating hormone and adrenocorticotropin concentrations in response to thyrotropin-releasing hormone and comparison with adrenocorticotropin concentration after domperidone administration in healthy horses and horses with pituitary pars intermedia dysfunction / J. Beech, D. McFarlane, S. Lindborg (et al.), *J Am Vet Med Assoc* 238 (2011): 1305–1315

10. Antinociceptive effects, acute toxicity and chemical composition of Vitex agnus-castus essential oil / E. Khalilzadeh, G. Vafaei Saiah, H. Hasannejad (et al.), *Avicenna J Phytomed* 5 (2015): 218–230

11. Antioxidant nutrients : a systematic review of trace elements and vitamins in the critically ill patient / D. Heyland, R. Dhaliwal, U. Suchner (et al.), *Intensive Care Med* 31 (2005): 327–337

12. Assessment of tissue-specific cortisol activity with regard to degeneration of the suspensory ligaments in horses with pituitary pars intermedia dysfunction / S. Hofberger, F. Gauff, D. Thaller (et al.), *Am J Vet Res* 79 (2018): 199–210

13. Association between hyperinsulinaemia and laminitis severity at the time of pituitary pars intermedia dysfunction diagnosis / E. Tadros, J. Fowlie, K. Refsal (et al.), *Equine Vet J* 51 (2019): 52–56

14. Association of season and pasture grazing with blood hormone and metabolite concentrations in horses with presumed pituitary pars intermedia dysfunction / N. Frank, S. Elliott, K. Chameroy (et al.), *J Vet Intern Med* 24 (2010): 1167–1175

15. Beta-endorphin stimulates corticosterone synthesis in isolated rat adrenal cells / G. Shanker, R. Sharma, *Biochem Biophys Res Commun* 86 (1979): 1–5

16. Bioactive and immunoreactive adrenocorticotropin in normal equine pituitary and in pituitary tumors of horses with Cushing's disease / D. Orth, W. Nicholson, *Endocrinology* 111 (1982): 559–563

17. Bioactivity of plasma ACTH from PPID-affected horses compared to normal horses / M. Cordero, B. Shrauner, D. McFarlane, *J Vet Intern Med* 25 (2011): 664

18. Biochemical indices of vascular function, glucose metabolism and oxidative stress in horses with equine Cushing's disease / J. Keen, M. McLaren, K. Chandler (et al.), *Equine Vet J* 36 (2004): 226–229

19. Can endocrine dysfunction be reliably tested in aged horses that are experiencing pain? / H. Gehlen, N. Jaburg, R. Merle (et al.), *Animals* 10 (2020): 1426

20. Carbonyl reductase 1 catalyzes 20β-reduction of glucocorticoids, modulating receptor activation and metabolic complications of obesity / R. Morgan, K. Beck, M. Nixon (et al.), *Sci Rep* 7 (2017): 10633

21. Central melanocortin receptors regulate insulin action / S. Obici, Z. Feng, J. Tan (et al.), *J Clin Invest* 108 (2001): 1079–1085

22. Changes in proportions of dry matter intakes by ponies with access to pasture and haylage for 3 and 20 hours per day respectively, for six weeks / J. Ince, A. Longland, C. Newbold (et al.), *J Equine Vet Sci* 31 (2011): 283–283

23. Chromium propionate increases insulin sensitivity in horses following oral and intravenous carbohydrate administration / J. Spears, K. Lloyd, P. Siciliano (et al.), *J Anim Sci* 98 (2020): skaa095

24. Chronic stress and age-related increases in the proinflammatory cytokine IL-6 / J. Kiecolt-Glaser, K. Preacher, R. MacCallum (et al.), In: *Proc. of the National Academy of Sciences* 100 (2003): 9090–9095

25. Circadian and circannual rhythms of cortisol, ACTH, and α-melanocyte-stimulating hormone in healthy horses / M. Cordero, B. Brorsen, D. McFarlane, *Domest Anim Endocrinol* 43 (2012): 317–324

26. Circannual variation in plasma adrenocorticotropic hormone concentrations in the UK in normal horses and ponies, and those with pituitary pars intermedia dysfunction / V. Copas, A. Durham, *Equine Vet J* 44 (2012): 440–443

27. Clinical implications of using adrenocorticotropic hormone diagnostic cutoffs or reference intervals to diagnose pituitary pars intermedia dysfunction in mature horses / R. Horn, A. Stewart, K. Jackson (et al.), *J Vet Intern Med* 35 (2021): 560–570

28. Clinical presentation, diagnosis, and prognosis of chronic laminitis in Europe / R. Eustace, *Vet Clin North Am Equine Pract* 26 (2010): 391–405

29. Clinically and temporally specific diagnostic thresholds for plasma ACTH in the horse / A. Durham, B. Clarke, J. Potier (et al.), *Equine Vet J* 53 (2021): 250–260

30. Comparison of cortisol and ACTH responses after administration of thyrotropin releasing hormone in normal horses and those with pituitary pars intermedia dysfunction / J. Beech, R. Boston, S. Lindborg, *J Vet Intern Med* 25 (2011): 1431–1438

31. Comparison of hair follicle histology between horses with pituitary pars intermedia dysfunction and excessive hair growth and normal aged horses / M. Innerå, A. Petersen, D. Desjardins (et al.), *Vet Dermatol* 24 (2013): 212–217

32. Comparison of owner-reported health problems with veterinary assessment of geriatric horses in the United Kingdom / J. Ireland, P. Clegg, C. McGowan (et al.), *Equine Vet J* 44 (2012): 94–100

33. Comparison of two diagnostic methods to detect insulin dysregulation in horses under field conditions / L. Van Den Wollenberg, V. Vandendriessche, K. van Maanen (et al.), *J Equine Vet Sci* 88 (2020): 102954

34. Comparison of two methods for measurement of equine adrenocorticotropin / H. Banse, N. Schultz, M. McCue (et al.), *J Vet Diagn Invest* 30 (2018): 233–237

35. Comparison of vitex agnus castus extract and pergolide in treatment of equine Cushing's syndrome / J. Beech, M. Donaldson, S. Lindborg, In: *Proc. of the 48th Annual Convention of the American Association of Equine Practitioners* (2002): 175–177

36. Continuous intravenous infusion of glucose induces endogenous hyperinsulinaemia and lamellar histopathology in Standardbred horses / M. de Laat, M. Sillence, C. McGowan (et al.), *Vet J* 191 (2012): 317–322

37. Correlation between plasma alpha-melanocyte-stimulating hormone concentration and body mass index in healthy horses / M. Donaldson, D. McFarlane, A. Jorgensen (et al.), *Am J Vet Res* 65 (2004): 1469–1473

38. Correlation of pituitary histomorphometry with adrenocorticotrophic hormone response to domperidone administration in the diagnosis of equine pituitary pars intermedia dysfunction / M. Miller, I. Pardo, L. Jackson (et al.), *Vet Pathol* 45 (2008): 26–38

39. Corticosteroid-associated laminitis / S. Bailey, *Vet Clin North Am Equine Pract* 26 (2010): 277–285

40. Cortisol, adrenocorticotropic hormone, serotonin, adrenaline and noradrenaline serum concentrations in relation to disease and stress in the horse / I. Ayala, N. Martos, G. Silvan (et al.), *Res Vet Sci* 93 (2012): 103–107

41. A cross-sectional study of geriatric horses in the United Kingdom. Part 2 : Health care and disease / J. Ireland, P. Clegg, C. McGowan (et al.), *Equine Vet J* 43 (2011): 37–44

42. A C-terminal HSP90 inhibitor restores glucocorticoid sensitivity and relieves a mouse allograft model of Cushing disease / M. Riebold, C. Kozany, L. Freiburger (et al.), *Nat Med* 21 (2015): 276–280

43. Curcumin (diferuloylmethane) inhibits cell proliferation, induces apoptosis, and decreases hormone levels and secretion in pituitary tumor cells / M. Miller, S. Chen, J. Woodliff (et al.), *Endocrinology* 149 (2008): 4158–4167

44. Cushing's disease : a new approach to therapy in equine and canine patients / M. Elliott, *Br Homeopath J* 90 (2001): 33–36

45. Cushing's syndromes, insulin resistance and endocrinopathic laminitis / P. Johnson, N. Messer, V. Ganjam, *Equine Vet J* 36 (2004): 194–198

46. Cyproheptadine and desmethylcyproheptadine directly inhibit the release of adrenocorticotrophin and beta-lipotrophin/beta-endorphin activity from the neurointermediate lobe of the rat pituitary gland / S. Lamberts, E. Bons, P. Uitterlinden (et al.), *J Endocrinol* 96 (1983): 395–400

47. Cytokine dysregulation in aged horses and horses with pituitary pars intermedia dysfunction / D. McFarlane, T. Holbrook *J Vet Intern Med* 22 (2008): 436–42

48. Diabetes, insulin resistance, and metabolic syndrome in horses / P. Johnson, C. Wiedmeyer, A. LaCarrubba (et al.), *J Diabetes Sci Technol* 6 (2012): 534–540

49. Diagnosis and treatment of hyperprolactinemia : an endocrine society clinical practice guideline / S. Melmed, F. Casanueva, A. Hoffman (et al.), *J Clin Endocrinol Metab* 96 (2011): 273–288

50. The diagnosis of equine insulin dysregulation / F. Bertin, M. de Laat, *Equine Vet J* 49 (2017): 570–576

51. Diagnostic frequency, response to therapy, and long-term prognosis among horses and ponies with pituitary par intermedia dysfunction, 1993-2004 / B. Rohrbach, J. Stafford, R. Clermont (et al.), *J Vet Intern Med* 26 (2012): 1027–1034

52. Diagnostic testing for equine endocrine diseases : confirmation versus confusion / D. McFarlane. *Vet Clin North Am Equine Pract* 35 (2019): 327–338

53. Diagnostic testing for pituitary pars intermedia dysfunction in horses / N. Dybdal, K. Hargreaves, J. Madigan (et al.), *J Am Vet Med Assoc* 204 (1994): 627–632

54. Dietary restriction in combination with a nutraceutical supplement for the management of equine metabolic syndrome in horses / C. McGowan, A. Dugdale, G. Pinchbeck (et al.), *Vet J* 196 (2013): 153–159

55. Dietary supplementation with short-chain fructo-oligosaccharides improves insulin sensitivity in obese horses / F. Respondek, K. Myers, T. Smith (et al.), *J Anim Sci* 89 (2011): 77–83

56. Does equine pituitary pars intermedia dysfunction (PPID) affect immune responses to vaccination? / Dorothy Russell Havemeyer Foundation, In: *Proc. of the 3rd Equine Endocrine Summit* (2014): 8

57. Does pergolide therapy prevent laminitis in horses diagnosed with pituitary pars intermedia dysfunction? / E. Knowles, *Equine Vet Educ* 31 (2019): 278–280

58. Dopamine-regulated adrenocorticotropic hormone secretion in lactating rats : functional plasticity of melanotropes / M. Oláh, P. Fehér, Z. Ihm (et al.), *Neuroendocrinology* 90 (2009): 391–401

59. Dysregulation of cortisol metabolism in equine pituitary pars intermedia dysfunction / R. Morgan, J. Keen, N. Homer (et al.), *Endocrinology* 159 (2018): 3791–3800

60. ECEIM consensus statement on equine metabolic syndrome / A. Durham, N. Frank, C. McGowan (et al.), *J Vet Intern Med* 33 (2019): 335–349

61. The effect of acute exercise on the secretion of corticotropin-releasing factor, arginine vasopressin, and adrenocorticotropin as measured in pituitary venous blood from the horse / S. Alexander, C. Irvine, M. Ellis (et al.), *Endocrinology* 128 (1991): 65–72

62. Effect of age, season, body condition, and endocrine status on serum free cortisol fraction and insulin concentration in horses / K. Hart, D. Wochele, N. Norton (et al.), *J Vet Intern Med* 30 (2016): 653–663

63. Effect of corticotropin-like intermediate lobe peptide on pancreatic exocrine function in isolated rat pancreatic lobules. / J. Marshall, L. Kapcala, L. Manning (et al.), *J Clin Invest* 74 (1984): 1886–1889

64. The effect of curcumin supplementation on circulating adiponectin: a systematic review and meta-analysis of randomized controlled trials / C. Clark, E. Ghaedi, A. Arab (et al.), *Diabetes Metab Syndr* 13 (2019): 2819–2825

65. Effect of dietary carbohydrates and time of year on ACTH and cortisol concentrations in adult and aged horses / S. Jacob, R. Geor, P. Weber (et al.), *Domest Anim Endocrinol* 63 (2018): 15–22

66. The effect of equine metabolic syndrome on the ovarian follicular environment / D. Sessions-Bresnahan, E. Carnevale, *J Anim Sci* 92 (2014): 1485–1494

67. The effect of exercise on plasma concentrations of inflammatory markers in normal and previously laminitic ponies / N. Menzies-Gow, H. Wray, S. Bailey (et al.), *Equine Vet J* 46 (2014): 317–321

68. The effect of geographic location, breed, and pituitary dysfunction on seasonal adrenocorticotropin and α-melanocyte-stimulating hormone plasma concentrations in horses / D. McFarlane, M. Paradis, D. Zimmel (et al.), *J Vet Intern Med* 25 (2011): 872–881

69. Effect of hay soaking duration on metabolizable energy, total and prececal digestible crude protein and amino acids, non-starch carbohydrates, macronutrients and trace elements / M. Bochnia, C. Pietsch, M. Wensch-Dorendorf (et al.), *J Equine Vet Sci* 101 (2021): 103452

70. Effect of increased adiposity on insulin sensitivity and adipokine concentrations in horses and ponies fed a high fat diet, with or without a once daily high glycaemic meal / N. Bamford, S. Potter, P. Harris (et al.), *Equine Vet J* 48 (2016): 368–373

71. The effect of month and breed on plasma adrenocorticotropic hormone concentrations in equids / A. Durham, J. Potier, L. Huber, *Vet J* 286 (2022): 105857

72. The effect of long-term exercise on glucose metabolism and peripheral insulin sensitivity in standardbred horses / E. de Graaf-Roelfsema, M. van Ginneken, E. van Breda (et al.), *Equine Vet J* Suppl (2006): 221–225

73. The effect of oral metformin on insulin sensitivity in insulin-resistant ponies / K. Tinworth, R. Boston, P. Harris (et al.), *Vet J* 191 (2012): 79–84

74. The effect of season on the histologic and histomorphometric appearance of the equine pituitary gland / M. Cordero, D. McFarlane, M. Breshears (et al.), *J Equine Vet Sci* 32 (2012): 75–79

75. The effects of a special Agnus castus extract (BP1095E1) on prolactin secretion in healthy male subjects / P. Merz, C. Gorkow, A. Schrödter (et al.) *Exp Clin Endocrinol Diabetes* 104 (1996): 447–453

76. Effects of bromocriptine on glucose and insulin dynamics in normal and insulin dysregulated horses / C. Loos, K. Urschel, E. Vanzant (et al.) *Front Vet Sci* 9 (2022): 889888

77. Effects of a supplement containing chromium and magnesium on morphometric measurements, resting glucose, insulin concentrations and insulin sensitivity in laminitic obese horses / K. Chameroy, N. Frank, S. Elliott (et al.), *Equine Vet J* 43 (2011): 494–9

78. Effects of advanced age and pituitary pars intermedia dysfunction on components of the acute phase reaction in horses / A. Zak, N. Siwinska, S. Elzinga (et al.), *Domest Anim Endocrinol* 72 (2020): 106476

79. Effects of age and diet on glucose and insulin dynamics in the horse / J. Rapson, H. Schott, B. Nielsen (et al.), *Equine Vet J* 50 (2018): 690–696

80. Effects of common equine endocrine diseases on reproduction / T. Burns, *Vet Clin North Am Equine Pract* 32 (2016): 435–449

81. Effects of curcuma longa (turmeric) on postprandial plasma glucose and insulin in healthy subjects / J. Wickenberg, S. Ingemansson, J. Hlebowicz, *Nutr J* 9 (2010): 43

82. The effects of curcumin on diabetes mellitus: a systematic review / L. Marton, L. Pescinini, M. Camargo (et al), *Front Endocrinol* 12 (2021): 669448

83. Effects of diet-induced weight gain on insulin sensitivity and plasma hormone and lipid concentrations in horses / R. Carter, L. McCutcheon, L. George (et al.), *Am J Vet Res* 70 (2009): 1250–1258

84. Effects of docosahexaenoic acid (DHA)-rich microalgae supplementation on metabolic and inflammatory parameters in horses with equine metabolic syndrome / S. Elzinga, A. Betancourt, C. Stewart (et al.), *J Equine Vet Sci* 83 (2019): 102811

85. Effects of exercise training on adiposity, insulin sensitivity, and plasma hormone and lipid concentrations in overweight or obese, insulin-resistant horses / R. Carter, L. McCutcheon, E. Valle (et al.), *Am J Vet Res* 71 (2010): 314–321

86. Effects of incretin hormones on beta-cell mass and function, body weight, and hepatic and myocardial function / S. Mudaliar, R. Henry, *Am J Med* 123 (2010): 19–27

87. Effects of oral administration of levothyroxine sodium on serum concentrations of thyroid gland hormones and responses to injections of thyrotropin-releasing hormone in healthy adult mares / C. Sommardahl, N. Frank, S. Elliott (et al.), *Am J Vet Res* 66 (2005): 1025–1031

88. Effects of the insulin-sensitizing drug pioglitazone and lipopolysaccharide administration on insulin sensitivity in horses / J. Suagee, B. Corl, J. Wearn (et al.), *J Vet Intern Med* 25 (2011): 356–364

89. Effects of pituitary pars intermedia dysfunction and Prascend (pergolide tablets) treatment on endocrine and immune function in horses / A. Miller, A. Loynachan, H. Bush (et al.), *Domest Anim Endocrinol* 74 (2021): 106531

90. Effects of pretreatment with dexamethasone or levothyroxine sodium on endotoxin-induced alterations in glucose and insulin dynamics in horses / F. Tóth, N. Frank, R. Geor (et al.), *Am J Vet Res* 71 (2010): 60–68

91. Effects of soaking on the water-soluble carbohydrate and crude protein content of hay / A. Longland, C. Barfoot, P. Harris, *Vet Rec* 168 (2011): 618

92. Effects of the multi-compound complex in Corticosal in 177 horses with PPID in a retrospective veterinary questionnaire analysis in Germany / E. Schramm, A. Schwarz, H. Alber (et al.), *Pferdeheilkunde* 34 (2018): 538–549

93. The effect of trailering and dentistry on resting adrenocorticotropic hormone concentration in horses / J. Haffner, R. Hoffman, S. Grubbs, In: *Proc. of the 4th Global Equine Endocrine Symposium* (2020): 13

94. Efficacy of a novel palatable pergolide paste formulation for the treatment of pituitary pars intermedia dysfunction (PPID) in ponies / I. N. Maisonpierre, M. Sutton, *Equine Vet J* 50 (2018): 12–13

95. Efficacy of pergolide for the management of equine pituitary pars intermedia dysfunction : a systematic review / R. Tatum, C. McGowan, J. Ireland, *Vet J* 266 (2020): 105562

96. Efficacy of trilostane for the treatment of equine Cushing's syndrome / C. McGowan, R. Neiger, *Equine Vet J* 35 (2003): 414–418

97. Endocrine and metabolic dysregulation in laminitis: role of pituitary dysfunction / P. Johnson In: *Equine Laminitis* (2017): 134–140

98. Endocrine disease in aged horses / A. Durham, *Vet Clin North Am Equine Pract* 32 (2016): 301–315

99. Endocrine disorders and laminitis / E. Tadros, N. Frank, *Equine Vet Educ* 25 (2013): 152–162

100. Endocrine disorders of the equine athlete / N. Frank, *Vet Clin North Am Equine Pract* 34 (2018): 299–312

101. Endocrinopathic laminitis / N. Grenager, *Vet Clin North Am Equine Pract* 37 (2021): 619–638

102. Epidemiology of pituitary pars intermedia dysfunction : a systematic literature review of clinical presentation, disease prevalence and risk factors / J. Ireland, C. McGowan, *Vet J* 235 (2018): 22–33

103. Equine cushing-like syndrome: diagnosis and therapy in two cases / M. Sgorbini, D. Panzani, M. Maccheroni (et al.), *Vet Res Commun* 28 Suppl 1 (2004): 377–380

104. Equine Cushing's disease / P. McCue, *Vet Clin North Am Equine Pract* 18 (2002): 533–543

105. Equine Cushing's disease : differential regulation of beta-endorphin processing in tumors of the intermediate pituitary / W. Millington, N. Dybdal, R. Dawson (et al.), *Endocrinology* 123 (1988): 1598–1604

106. Equine Cushing's disease : plasma immunoreactive proopiolipomelanocortin peptide and cortisol levels basally and in response to diagnostic tests / D. Orth, M. Holscher, M. Wilson (et al.), *Endocrinology* 110 (1982): 1430–1441

107. Equine hyperlipidemias / H. McKenzie, *Vet Clin North Am Equine Pract* 27 (2011): 59–72

108. Equine insulin receptor and insulin-like growth factor-1 receptor expression in digital lamellar tissue and insulin target tissues / A. Kullmann, P. Weber, J. Bishop (et al.), *Equine Vet J* 48 (2016): 626–632

109. Equine laminitis: induced by 48 h hyperinsulinaemia in Standardbred horses / M. de Laat, C. McGowan, M. Sillence (et al.) *Equine Vet J* 42 (2010): 129–135

110. Equine laminitis: ultrastructural lesions detected in ponies following hyperinsulinaemia / A. Nourian, K. Asplin, C. McGowan (et al.), *Equine Vet J* 41 (2009): 671–677

111. Equine metabolic syndrome / N. Frank, R. Geor, S. Bailey (et al.), *J Vet Intern Med* 24 (2010): 467–475

112. Equine metabolic syndrome / N. Frank, *Vet Clin North Am Equine Pract* 27 (2011): 73–92

113. Equine metabolic syndrome in UK native ponies and cobs is highly prevalent with modifiable risk factors / H. Carslake, G. Pinchbeck, C. Mcgowan, *Equine Vet J* (2020): 923–934

114. The equine metabolic syndrome peripheral Cushing's syndrome / P. Johnson, *Vet Clin North Am Equine Pract* 18 (2002): 271–293

115. Equine metabool syndroom / P. Deprez, *Vlaams Diergeneeskundig Tijdschrift* 88 (2019): 113–120

116. Equine pituitary neoplasia : a clinical report of 21 cases (1990-1992) / J. van der Kolk, H. Kalsbeek, E. van Garderen (et al.), *Vet Rec* 133 (1993): 594–597

117. Equine pituitary pars intermedia dysfunction / D. McFarlane, *Vet Clin North Am Equine Pract* 27 (2011): 93–113

118. Equine pituitary pars intermedia dysfunction : a spontaneous model of synucleinopathy / J. Fortin, A. Hetak, K. Duggan (et al.), *Sci Rep* 11 (2021): 16036

119. Equine pituitary pars intermedia dysfunction : current perspectives on diagnosis and management / C. Spelta, *Vet Med (Auckl)* 6 (2015): 293–300

120. Equine pituitary pars intermedia dysfunction : current understanding and recommendations from the Australian and New Zealand Equine Endocrine Group / C. Secombe, S. Bailey, M. de Laat (et al.), *Aust Vet J* 96 (2018): 233–242

121. Evaluation of basal plasma alpha-melanocyte-stimulating hormone and adrenocorticotrophic hormone concentrations for the diagnosis of pituitary pars intermedia dysfunction from a population of aged horses / T. McGowan, G. Pinchbeck, C. McGowan, *Equine Vet J* 45 (2013): 66–73

122. Evaluation of combined testing to simultaneously diagnose pituitary pars intermedia dysfunction and insulin dysregulation in horses / R. Horn, F. Bertin, *J Vet Intern Med* 33 (2019): 2249–2256

123. Evaluation of dynamic testing for pituitary pars intermedia dysfunction diagnosis in donkeys / S. Mejia-Pereira, A. Perez-Ecija, B. Buchanan (et al.), *Equine Vet J* 51 (2019): 481–488

124. Evaluation of genetic and metabolic predispositions and nutritional risk factors for pasture-associated laminitis in ponies / K. Treiber, D. Kronfeld, T. Hess (et al.), *J Am Vet Med Assoc* 228 (2006): 1538–1545

125. Evaluation of plasma ACTH, alpha-melanocyte-stimulating hormone, and insulin concentrations during various photoperiods in clinically normal horses and ponies and those with pituitary pars intermedia dysfunction / J. Beech, R. Boston, D. McFarlane (et al.), *J Am Vet Med Assoc* 235 (2009): 715–722

126. Evaluation of suspected pituitary pars intermedia dysfunction in horses with laminitis / M. Donaldson, A. Jorgensen, J. Beech, *J Am Vet Med Assoc* 224 (2004): 1123–1127

127. Evaluation of the effects of age and pituitary pars intermedia dysfunction on corneal sensitivity in horses / C. Miller, M. Utter, J. Beech, *Am J Vet Res* 74 (2013): 1030–1035

128. Exercise-induced alterations in plasma concentrations of ghrelin, adiponectin, leptin, glucose, insulin, and cortisol in horses / M. Gordon, K. McKeever, C. Betros (et al.), *Vet J* 173 (2007): 532–540

129. Exposure to glyphosate- and/or mn/zn-ethylene-bis-dithiocarbamate-containing pesticides leads to degeneration of γ-aminobutyric acid and dopamine neurons in caenorhabditis elegans / R. Negga, J. Stuart, M. Machen (et al.), *Neurotox Res* 21 (2012): 281–290

130. Extrapituitary and pituitary pathological findings in horses with pituitary pars intermedia dysfunction : a retrospective study / C. Glover, L. Miller, N. Dybdal (et al.), *J Equine Vet Sci* 29 (2009): 146–153

131. Factors associated with survival, laminitis and insulin dysregulation in horses diagnosed with equine pituitary pars intermedia dysfunction / R. Horn, N. Bamford, T. Afonso (et al.), *Equine Vet J* 51 (2019): 440–445

132. Fecal egg counts after anthelmintic administration to aged horses and horses with pituitary pars intermedia dysfunction / D. McFarlane, G. Hale, E. Johnson (et al.), *J Am Vet Med Assoc* 236 (2010): 330–334

133. Genetics of equine endocrine and metabolic disease / E. Norton, M. McCue, *Vet Clin North Am Equine Pract* 36 (2020): 341–352

134. Glucocorticoid receptor immunoreactivity in the rat intermediate lobe / L. Bertini, M. Westphal, R. Kloet (et al.), *J Neuroendocrinol* 1 (1989): 465–471

135. Glucocorticoids and laminitis in horses / P. Johnson, N. Messer, D. Bowles (et al.), *Compendium on Continuing Education for the Practising Veterinarian* 26 (2004): 547–558

136. Glucocorticoids, metabolism and metabolic diseases / A. Vegiopoulos, S. Herzig, *Mol Cell Endocrinol* 275 (2007): 43–61

137. Glucose tolerance and insulin sensitivity in ponies and Standardbred horses / L. Jeffcott, J. Field, J. McLean (et al.), *Equine Vet J* 18 (1986): 97–101

138. The gut microbiome of horses : current research on equine enteral microbiota and future perspectives / A. Kauter, L. Epping, T. Semmler (et al.), *Anim Microbiome* 1 (2019): 14

139. Heritability of metabolic traits associated with equine metabolic syndrome in Welsh ponies and Morgan horses / E. Norton, N. Schultz, A. Rendahl (et al.), *Equine Vet J* 51 (2019): 475–480

140. Horse-factors influencing the seasonal increase in plasma acth secretion / A. Durham, In: *Proc. of the International Equine Endocrinology Summit by Havemeyer Foundation* (2017): 36–37

141. How does Cushing's disease relate to laminitis? : advances in diagnosis and treatment / N. Grenager, *J Equine Vet Sci* 30 (2010): 482–490

142. Hyperinsulinaemia increases vascular resistance and endothelin-1 expression in the equine digit / F. Gauff, B. Patan-Zugaj, T. Licka, *Equine Vet J* 45 (2013): 613–618

143. Hypothalamic-pituitary gland axis function and dysfunction in horses / S. Hurcombe, *Vet Clin North Am Equine Pract* 27 (2011): 1–17

144. Immune dysfunction in aged horses / D. McFarlane, *Vet Clin North Am Equine Pract* 32 (2016): 333–341

145. Immunocytochemical demonstration of proopiomelanocortin-derived peptides in pituitary adenomas of the pars intermedia in horses / M. Heinrichs, W. Baumgärtner, C. Capen, *Vet Pathol* 27 (1990): 419–425

146. Immunocytochemical localization of adrenocorticotropic hormone-immunoreactive cells of the pars intermedia in thoroughbreds / T. Okada, T. Shimomuro, M. Oikawa (et al.), *Am J Vet Res* 58 (1997): 920–924

147. Immunosenescence in horses / D. McFarlane, In: Proc. of the 59th Annual Convention of the American Association of Equine Practitioners (2013) 316

148. Improved insulin sensitivity in hyperinsulinaemic ponies through physical conditioning and controlled feed intake / J. Freestone, R. Beadle, K. Shoemaker (et al.), *Equine Vet J* 24 (1992): 187–190

149. An in vitro model of Parkinson's disease : linking mitochondrial impairment to altered alpha-synuclein metabolism and oxidative damage / T. Sherer, R. Betarbet, A. Stout (et al.), *J Neurosci* 22 (2002): 7006–7015

150. Inducing weight loss in native ponies : is straw a viable alternative to hay? / M. Dosi, R. Kirton, S. Hallsworth (et al.), *Vet Rec* 187 (2020): 60

151. Induction of laminitis by prolonged hyperinsulinaemia in clinically normal ponies / K. Asplin, M. Sillence, C. Pollitt (et al.), *Vet J* 174 (2007): 530–535

152. Inflammation, oxidative stress, and obesity / A. Fernández-Sánchez, E. Madrigal-Santillán, M. Bautista (et al.), *Int J Mol Sci* 12 (2011): 3117–3132

153. Inflammation: the common pathway of stress-related diseases / Y. Liu, Y. Wang, C. Jiang, *Front Hum Neurosci* 11 (2017): 316

154. Influence of dietary restriction and low-intensity exercise on weight loss and insulin sensitivity in obese equids / N. Bamford, S. Potter, C. Baskerville (et al.), *J Vet Intern Med* 33 (2019): 280–286

155. Influence of feeding status, time of the day, and season on baseline adrenocorticotropic hormone and the response to thyrotropin releasing hormone-stimulation test in healthy horses / E. Diez de Castro, I. Lopez, B. Cortes (et al.), *Domest Anim Endocrinol* 48 (2014): 77–83

156. Insulin dysregulation / N. Frank, E. Tadros, *Equine Vet J* 46 (2014): 103–112

157. Insulin resistance and hyperinsulinemia: is hyperinsulinemia the cart or the horse? / M. Shanik, Y. Xu, J. Skrha (et al.), *Diabetes Care* 31 (2008): S262-268

158. Insulinaemic and glycaemic responses to three forages in ponies / H. Carslake, C. Argo, G. Pinchbeck (et al.), *Vet J* 235 (2018): 83–89

159. Intravenous injection of insulin for measuring insulin sensitivity in horses : effects of epinephrine, feeding regimen, and supplementation with cinnamon for fish oil / L. Earl, *LSU Master's Theses 4144* (2011)

160. Investigation of rhythms of secretion and repeatability of plasma adrenocorticotropic hormone concentrations in healthy horses and horses with pituitary pars intermedia dysfunction / D. Rendle, E. Litchfield, J. Heller (et al.), *Equine Vet J* 46 (2014): 113–117

161. Involvement of constitutive (COX-1) and inducible cyclooxygenase (COX-2) in the adrenergic-induced ACTH and corticosterone secretion / J. Bugajski, R. Głód, A. Gadek-Michalska (et al.), *J Physiol Pharmacol* 52 (2001): 795–809

162. Is cinnamon efficacious for glycaemic control in type-2 diabetes mellitus? / S. Sharma, A. Mandal, R. Kant (e t al.), *J Pak Med Assoc* 70 (2020): 2065–2069

163. Lamellar pathology in horses with pituitary pars intermedia dysfunction / N. Karikoski, J. Patterson-Kane, E. Singer (et al.), *Equine Vet J* 48 (2016): 472–478

164. Laminitis and the equine metabolic syndrome / P. Johnson, C. Wiedmeyer, A. LaCarrubba (et al.), *Vet Clin North Am Equine Pract* 26 (2010): 239–255

165. Laminitis trust clinical trial using vitex in equine cushing's disease / R. Eustace

166. Localisation of 11 beta-hydroxysteroid dehydrogenase-tissue specific protector of the mineralocorticoid receptor / C. Edwards, P. Stewart, D. Burt (et al.), *Lancet* 2 (1988): 986–989

167. Long-term and short-term dopaminergic (cabergoline) and antidopaminergic (sulpiride) effects on insulin response to glucose, glucose response to insulin, or both, in horses / N. Arana Valencia, D. Thompson, E. Oberhaus, *J Equine Vet Sci* 59 (2017): 95–103

168. Long-term response of equids with pituitary pars intermedia dysfunction to treatment with pergolide / H. Schott, H. Rapson, J. Marteniuk (et al.), In: *Proc. of the 60th Annual Convention of the American Association of Equine Practitioners* (2014): 329

169. Markers of muscle atrophy and impact of treatment with pergolide in horses with pituitary pars intermedia dysfunction and muscle atrophy / H. Banse, A. Whitehead, D. McFarlane (et al.), *Domest Anim Endocrinol* 76 (2021): 106620

170. Measurement of C-peptide concentrations and responses to somatostatin, glucose infusion, and insulin resistance in horses / F. Tóth, N. Frank, T. Martin-Jiménez (et al.), *Equine Vet J* 42 (2010): 149–155

171. Mechanisms linking glucose homeostasis and iron metabolism toward the onset and progression of type 2 diabetes / J. Fernández-Real, D. McClain, M. Manco, *Diabetes Care* 38 (2015): 2169–2176

172. The Michigan Cushing's project / H. Scott, C. Coursen, S. Eberhart, In: *Proc. of the 47th Annual Convention of the American Association of Equine Practitioners* (2001): 22–24

173. Mitochondrial dysfunction and oxidative stress in neurodegenerative diseases / M. Lin, M. Beal, *Nature* 443 (2006): 787–795

174. Moderate dietary carbohydrate improves and high dietary fat impairs glucose tolerance in aged thoroughbred geldings / J. Pagan, In: *Proc. of the Australasian Equine Science Symposium* (2012): 20

175. A 'modified Obel' method for the severity scoring of (endocrinopathic) equine laminitis / A. Meier, M. de Laat, C. Pollitt (et al.), *PeerJ* 7 (2019): 7084

176. Mucuna pruriens in Parkinson disease: a double-blind, randomized, controlled, crossover study / R. Cilia, J. Laguna, E. Cassani (et al.), *Neurology* 89 (2017): 432–438

177. Nitration and increased alpha-synuclein expression associated with dopaminergic neurodegeneration in equine pituitary pars intermedia dysfunction / D. McFarlane, N. Dybdal, M.Donaldson (et al.), *J Neuroendocrinol* 17 (2005): 73–80

178. A novel technique for measuring hypothalamic and pituitary hormone secretion rates from collection of pituitary venous effluent in the normal horse / C. Irvine, S. Alexander, *J Endocrinol* 113 (1987): 183–192

179. Nutritional considerations when dealing with an obese adult equine / M. Shepherd, P. Harris, K. Martinson, *Vet Clin North Am Equine Pract* 37 (2021): 111–137

180. Nutritional considerations when dealing with an underweight adult or senior horse / N. Jarvis, H. McKenzie, *Vet Clin North Am Equine Pract* 37 (2021): 89–110

181. Nutritional management of the older horse / C.McG. Argo, *Vet Clin North Am Equine Pract* 32 (2016): 343–354

182. Obesity and corticosteroids: 11beta-hydroxysteroid type 1 as a cause and therapeutic target in metabolic disease / N. Morton, *Mol Cell Endocrinol* 316 (2010): 154–164

183. Occupational exposures and neurodegenerative diseases : a systematic literature review and meta-analyses / L. Gunnarsson, L. Bodin, *Int J Environ Res Public Health* 16 (2019): 337

184. Oral supplementation of magnesium aspartate hydrochloride in horses with Equine Metabolic Syndrome / H. Gehlen, J. Winter, R. Merle (et al.), *Pferdeheilkunde* 32 (2016): 372–377

185. Oxidative stress / C. Soffler, *Vet Clin North Am Equine Pract* 23 (2007): 135–157

186. Oxidative stress induced-neurodegenerative diseases : the need for antioxidants that penetrate the blood brain barrier / Y. Gilgun-Sherki, E. Melamed, D. Offen, *Neuropharmacology* 40 (2001): 959–975

187. Paradigm shifts in understanding equine laminitis / J. Patterson-Kane, N. Karikoski, C. McGowan, *Vet J* 231 (2018): 33–40

188. Pasture nonstructural carbohydrates and equine laminitis / A. Longland, B. Byrd, *J Nutr* 136 (2006): 2099S–2102S

189. Pathology of natural cases of equine endocrinopathic laminitis associated with hyperinsulinemia / N. Karikoski, C. McGowan, E. Singer (et al.), *Vet Pathol* 52 (2015): 945–956

190. Pathophysiology and clinical features of pituitary pars intermedia dysfunction / D. McFarlane, *Equine Vet Educ* 26 (2014): 592–598

191. Pergolide protects dopaminergic neurons in primary culture under stress conditions / G. Gille, W. Rausch, S. Hung (et al.), *J Neural Transm* (Vienna) 109 (2002): 633–643

192. Pharmacokinetics and bioavailability of metformin in horses / J. Hustace, A. Firshman, J. Mata, *Am J Vet Res* 70 (2009): 665–668

193. Pharmacokinetic and pharmacodynamic properties of pergolide mesylate following long-term administration to horses with pituitary pars intermedia dysfunction / D. McFarlane, H. Banse, H. Knych (et al.), *J Vet Pharmacol Ther* 40 (2017): 158–164

194. Pharmacokinetics and pharmacodynamics of pergolide mesylate after oral administration in horses with pituitary pars intermedia dysfunction / D. Rendle, G. Doran, J. Ireland (et al.), *Domest Anim Endocrinol* 68 (2019): 135–141

195. The pharmacologic basis for the treatment of endocrinopathic laminitis / A. Durham, *Vet Clin North Am Equine Pract* 26 (2010): 303–314

196. Pituitary gland neuroendocrinology / P. Malven, In: *Proc. of the 15th Annual Forum of the American College of Veterinary Internal Medicine* (1997): 462–467

197. Pituitary pars intermedia dysfunction / D. McFarlane, P. Johnson, H. Schott, In: *Equine Laminitis* (2017): 334–340

198. Pituitary pars intermedia dysfunction / N. Frank, In: *Robinson's Current Therapy in Equine Medicine, 7th ed.* (2015): 574–575

199. Pituitary pars intermedia dysfunction and metabolic syndrome in donkeys / H. Gehlen, B. Schwarz, C. Bartmann (et al.), *Animals (Basel)* 10 (2020): 2335

200. Pituitary pars intermedia dysfunction bij het paard : belangrijke aandachtspunten en recente ontwikkelingen / B. Broux, L. Lefere, G. van Loon, *Vlaams Diergeneeskundig Tijdschrift* 82 (2013): 44

201. Pituitary pars intermedia dysfunction : diagnosis and treatment / A. Durham, C. Mcgowan, K. Fey (et al.), *Equine Vet Educ* 26 (2014): 216–223

202. Pituitary pars intermedia dysfunction does not necessarily impair insulin sensitivity in old horses / L. Mastro, A. Adams, K. Urschel, *Domest Anim Endocrinol* 50 (2015): 14–25

203. Pituitary pars intermedia dysfunction : equine Cushing's disease / H. Schott, *Vet Clin North Am Equine Pract* 18 (2002): 237–270

204. Pituitary pars intermedia dysfunction in the horse. Part II : diagnosis and treatment. / N. Dybdal, M. Levy, In: *Proc. of the 15th Annual Forum of the American College of Veterinary Internal Medicine* (1997): 470–472

205. Pituitary-independent Cushing's syndrome in a horse / J. van der Kolk, J. IJzer, P. Overgaauw (et al.), *Equine Vet J* 33 (2001): 110–112

206. Plasma steroid profiles before and after ACTH stimulation test in healthy horses / A. Kirchmeier, A. van Herwaarden, J. van der Kolk (et al.), *Domest Anim Endocrinol* 72 (2020): 106419

207. Polyuria and polydipsia in horses / E. McKenzie, *Vet Clin North Am Equine Pract* 23 (2007): 641–653

208. A potential link between insulin resistance and iron overload disorder in browsing rhinoceroses investigated through the use of an equine model / B. Nielsen, M. Vick, P. Dennis, *J Zoo Wildl Med* 43 (2012): 61–65

209. A potential role for lamellar insulin-like growth factor-1 receptor in the pathogenesis of hyperinsulinaemic laminitis / M. de Laat, C. Pollitt, M. Kyaw-Tanner (et al.), *Vet J* 197 (2013): 302–306

210. Prediction of incipient pasture-associated laminitis from hyperinsulinaemia, hyperleptinaemia and generalised and localised obesity in a cohort of ponies / R. Carter, K. Treiber, R. Geor (et al.), *Equine Vet J* 41 (2009): 171–178

211. Prevalence and analysis of equine periodontal disease, diastemata and peripheral caries in a first-opinion horse population in the UK / H. Nuttall, P. Ravenhill, *Vet J* 246 (2019): 98–102

212. Prevalence and risk factors for hyperinsulinaemia in ponies in Queensland, Australia / R. Morgan, T. McGowan, C. McGowan, *Aust Vet J* 92 (2014): 101–106

213. The prevalence of endocrinopathic laminitis among horses presented for laminitis at a first-opinion/referral equine hospital / N. Karikoski, I. Horn, T. McGowan (et al.), *Domest Anim Endocrinol* 41 (2011): 111–117

214. Prevalence, risk factors and clinical signs predictive for equine pituitary pars intermedia dysfunction in aged horses / T. Mcgowan, G. Pinchbeck, C. Mcgowan, *Equine Vet J* 45 (2013): 74–79

215. Prevalence, survival analysis and multimorbidity of chronic diseases in the general veterinarian-attended horse population of the UK / C. Welsh, M. Duz, T. Parkin (et al.), *Prev Vet Med* 131 (2016): 137–145

216. Proconvulsant potential of cyproheptadine in experimental animal models / D. Singh, R. Goel, *Fundam Clin Pharmacol* 24 (2010): 451–455

217. Profiles of pro-opiomelanocortin and encoded peptides, and their processing enzymes in equine pituitary pars intermedia dysfunction / J. Carmalt, S. Mortazavi, R. McOnie (et al.), *PLoS One* 13 (2018): e0190796

218. Proopiolipomelanocortin peptides in normal pituitary, pituitary tumor, and plasma of normal and Cushing's horses / M. Wilson, W. Nicholson, M. Holscher (et al.), *Endocrinology* 110 (1982): 941–954

219. Prospective cohort study evaluating risk factors for the development of pasture-associated laminitis in the United Kingdom / N. Menzies-Gow, P. Harris, J. Elliott, *Equine Vet J* 49 (2017): 300–306

220. Psyllium lowers blood glucose and insulin concentrations in horses / S. Moreaux, J. Nichols, J. Bowman (et al.), *J Equine Vet Sci* 31 (2011): 160–165

221. Rat intermediate lobe in culture : dopaminergic regulation of POMC biosynthesis and cell proliferation / D. Gehlert, J. Bishop, M. Schafer (et al.), *Peptides* 9 (1988): 161–168

222. Recommendations for the diagnosis and treatment of equine metabolic syndrome (EMS) / The Equine Endocrinology Group (2020)

223. Recommendations for the diagnosis and treatment of pituitary pars intermedia dysfunction (PPID) / The Equine Endocrinology Group (2021)

224. The regulation of muscle mass by endogenous glucocorticoids / T. Braun, D. Marks, *Front Physiol* 6 (2015): 12

225. Relationship between endogenous plasma adrenocorticotropic hormone concentration and reproductive performance in Thoroughbred broodmares / T. Tsuchiya, R. Noda, H. Ikeda (et al.), *J Vet Intern Med* 35 (2021): 2002–2008

226. Relationship between intracellular free magnesium concentration and the degree of insulin resistance in horses with equine metabolic syndrome / J. Winter, E. Müller, G. Sponder (et al.), *Pferdeheilkunde Equine Medicine* 36 (2020): 325–332

227. Relationships of inflamm-aging with circulating nutrient levels, body composition, age, and pituitary pars intermedia dysfunction in a senior horse population / M. Siard-Altman, P. Harris, A. Moffett-Krotky (et al.), *Vet Immunol Immunopathol* 221 (2020): 110013

228. Restoring pars intermedia dopamine concentrations and tyrosine hydroxylase expression levels with pergolide : evidence from horses with pituitary pars intermedia dysfunction / J. Fortin, M. Benskey, K. Lookingland (et al.), *BMC Vet Res* 16 (2020): 356

229. Results of a combined dexamethasone suppression/thyrotropin-releasing hormone stimulation test in healthy horses and horses suspected to have a pars intermedia pituitary adenoma / H. Eiler, J. Oliver, F. Andrews (et al.), *J Am Vet Med Assoc* 211 (1997): 79–81

230. The role of dopaminergic neurodegeneration in equine pituitary pars intermedia dysfunction (equine Cushing's disease). / D. McFarlane, M. Donaldson, T. Saleh (et al.), In: *Proc. of the 49th Annual Connvention of the American Association of Equine Practitioners* (2003): 233–237

231. Role of melanocortin in the long-term regulation of energy balance : lessons from a seasonal model / S. Schuhler, F. Ebling, *Peptides* 27 (2006): 301–309

232. The safety and efficacy in horses of certain nutraceuticals that claim to have health benefits / I. Vervuert, M. Stratton-Phelps, *Vet Clin North Am Equine Pract* 37 (2021): 207–222

233. Sarcopenia : characteristics, mechanisms and functional significance / M. Narici, N. Maffulli, *Br Med Bull* 95 (2010): 139–159

234. Seasonal changes in plasma adrenocorticotropic hormone and α-melanocyte-stimulating hormone in response to thyrotropin-releasing hormone in normal, aged horses / R. Funk, A. Stewart, A. Wooldridge (et al.), *J Vet Intern Med* 25 (2011): 579–585

235. Seasonal patterns of circulating β-endorphin, adrenocorticotropic hormone and cortisol levels in pregnant and barren mares. / E. Fazio, P. Medica, A. Ferlazzo, *Bulg J Vet Med* (2009): 125–135

236. Seasonal variation in serum concentrations of selected metabolic hormones in horses / N. Place, C. McGowan, S. Lamb (et al.), *J Vet Intern Med* 24 (2010): 650–654

237. Serum insulin concentrations in horses with equine Cushing's syndrome : response to a cortisol inhibitor and prognostic value / C. McGowan, R. Frost, D. Pfeiffer (et al.), *Equine Vet J* 36 (2004): 295–298

238. Spirulina platensis improves mitochondrial function impaired by elevated oxidative stress in adipose-derived mesenchymal stromal cells (ASCS) and intestinal epithelial cells (iecs), and enhances insulin sensitivity in equine metabolic syndrome (EMS) horses / D. Nawrocka, K. Kornicka, A. Śmieszek (et al.), *Mar Drugs* 15 (2017): 237

239. Spontaneous rupture of Achilles tendon: missed presentation of Cushing's syndrome / A. Mousa, S. Jones, A. Toft (et al.), *BMJ* 319 (1999): 560–561

240. Sulfur amino acids in Cushing's disease: insight in homocysteine and taurine levels in patients with active and cured disease / A. Faggiano, D. Melis, R. Alfieri (et al.), *J Clin Endocrinol Metab* 90 (2005): 6616–6622

241. Suspensory ligament degeneration associated with pituitary pars intermedia dysfunction in horses / S. Hofberger, F. Gauff, T. Licka, *Vet J* 203 (2015): 348–350

242. Sustained, low-intensity exercise achieved by a dynamic feeding system decreases body fat in ponies / M. de Laat, B. Hampson, M. Sillence (et al.), *J Vet Intern Med* 30 (2016): 1732–1738

243. Systemic and pituitary pars intermedia antioxidant capacity associated with pars intermedia oxidative stress and dysfunction in horses / D. McFarlane, A. Cribb, *Am J Vet Res* 66 (2005): 2065–2072

244. The oral glucose test predicts laminitis risk in ponies fed a diet high in nonstructural carbohydrates / A. Meier, M. de Laat, D. Reiche (et al.), *Domest Anim Endocrinol* 63 (2018): 1–9

245. Therapeutics for equine endocrine disorders / A. Durham, *Vet Clin North Am Equine Pract* 33 (2017): 127–139

246. Treatment of equine metabolic syndrome : a clinical case series / R. Morgan, J. Keen, C. McGowan, *Equine Vet J* 48 (2016): 422–426

247. Treatment with pergolide or cyproheptadine of pituitary pars intermedia dysfunction (equine Cushing's disease) / M. Donaldson, B. LaMonte, P. Morresey (et al.), *J Vet Intern Med* 16 (2002): 742–746

248. Update on equine odontoclastic tooth resorption and hypercementosis / L. Limone, *Vet Clin North Am Equine Pract* 36 (2020): 671–689

249. Use of the chasteberry preparation Corticosal for the treatment of pituitary pars intermedia dysfunction in horses / Z. Bradaric, A. May, H. Gehlen, *Pferdeheilkunde* 29 (2013): 721–728

250. Values for triglycerides, insulin, cortisol, and ACTH in a herd of normal donkeys / S. Dugat, T. Taylor, N. Matthews (et al.), *J Equine Vet Sci* 30 (2010): 141–144

251. Variation in plasma adrenocorticotropic hormone concentration and dexamethasone suppression test results with season, age, and sex in healthy ponies and horses / M. Donaldson, S. McDonnell, B. Schanbacher (et al.), *J Vet Intern Med* 19 (2005): 217–222

252. Vitamin B12-impaired metabolism produces apoptosis and Parkinson phenotype in rats expressing the transcobalamin-oleosin chimera in substantia nigra / C. Orozco-Barrios, S. Battaglia-Hsu, M. Arango-Rodriguez (et al.), *PLoS One* 4 (2009): 8268

253. Welfare, quality of life, and euthanasia of aged horses / C. McGowan, J. Ireland, *Vet Clin North Am Equine Pract* 32 (2016): 355–367

254. What's new in old horses? : postmortem diagnoses in mature and aged equids / M. Miller, G. Moore, F. Bertin (et al.), *Vet Pathol* 53 (2016): 390–398

255. Weight loss resistance: a further consideration for the nutritional management of obese equidae / C. Argo, G. Curtis, D. Grove-White (et al.), *Vet J* 194 (2012): 179–188

WEBSITES

- ecirhorse.org
- ker.com
- rossdales.com
- safergrass.org
- thehorse.com
- thelaminitissite.org
- vetfolio.com

PHOTOGRAPHERS

- Advanced Equine Therapies
- Anna Armbrust
- Barabara Trotman
- Cedric Coucke
- Christoph van Horst
- Classic Equine Equipment
- Cynthia Cooper
- David Selbert
- Donna Nyland
- Duplo
- Flash Dantz
- Jaqueline Verhagen
- Jiří Novák
- Kady Mauro
- Karin Schouwenburg
- Mandy Fontana
- Marsha Brouwer
- Michael Frank
- Michael Kesl
- Mirjam van Hoorn
- Mulography
- Myhre Equine Clinic
- Nikke de Kerf
- PaardEerlijk
- Pat Whelen
- Pavel Anoshin
- Pavel Šinkyrík
- Redwings Horse Sanctuary
- Robert Dlesk
- Rodnae Productions
- Rodolfo Quirós
- Royal Veterinary College, Londen
- Soft-ride
- University of Veterinary Medicine Hanover, Clinic for horses
- Valley Vet Supply
- Vladimír Motyčka
- W. Ellenberger
- Zefanja Vermeulen

GLOSSARY

Words that appear frequently in the text or that aren't further specified, are defined in the context of this book's subject. Definitions for italicised terms in the descriptions can be found elsewhere in the glossary.

ACTH
Adrenocorticotropic hormone. A *hormone* secreted by the *adenohypophysis*. Most of the ACTH in the intermediate lobe is converted into *alpha-MSH* and *CLIP*.

ADENOHYPOPHYSIS
Collective term for the anterior and intermediate lobe of the *pituitary gland*.

ADENOMA
Benign glandular tissue tumour.

ADIPOKINE
Hormone released by fat cells, that influences the immune system and appetite regulation, among other functions.

ADIPONECTIN
Adipokine that increases the body's *insulin* sensitivity.

ADIPOSITY
Type of overweight that is characterised by abnormal fat deposits and distribution.

ADRENAL ENLARGEMENT
Enlargement of the *adrenal glands* due to *hyperplasia* and *hypertrophy*.

ADRENAL GLANDS
Small hormone glands situated atop the kidneys.

ADRENALINE
Hormone and *neurotransmitter* that affects blood sugar levels, among other things.

ALPHA-MSH
Alpha-melanocyte-stimulating hormone. A *hormone* that is cleaved off from *ACTH*.

ANTIOXIDANT
A substance that reduces the oxidation of cells by *free radicals*.

BASEMENT MEMBRANE
Connective tissue that attaches the *dermal lamellae* to the *epidermal lamellae*.

BCS
Body Condition Score. Assessment system to classify body condition and fat deposition of horses.

BETA-ENDORPHIN
A *hormone* that is cleaved off from *POMC*.

BIOMARKER
A traceable substance introduced by a researcher, or a substance naturally present in the body that indicates a particular biological state or condition, such as antibodies demonstrating an infection.

BLOOD PLASMA
The liquid part of the blood, without the blood cells and platelets.

BLOOD SERUM
Bright yellow liquid obtained by allowing *blood plasma* to clot and then subjecting the clot to centrifugation.

CIRCADIAN RHYTHM
Biological cycle lasting approximately 24 hours, such as the human sleep-wake rhythm.

CLINICAL PICTURE
The overall presentation of objectively observable characteristics (*clinical signs*) associated with a disorder, syndrome or disease.

CLINICAL SIGN
A characteristic of a condition, which is objectively determinable.

CLIP
Corticotropin-like intermediate lobe peptide. A *hormone* that is cleaved off from *ACTH*.

CNS
Cresty Neck Score. Assessment system to classify neck circumference and thus overweight in horses.

CORTICOSTEROIDS
Hormones produced by the adrenal cortex, which can be categorised into *glucocorticoids* and mineralocorticoids. In the context of PPID, the primary involvement is with glucocorticoids.

CORTICOTROPE
Hormone-producing cell in the anterior lobe of the *pituitary gland*.

CORTISOL
Adrenal cortical hormone belonging to the *glucocorticoids*.

CORTISOL CLEARANCE
Breakdown and removal of *cortisol* from the body.

CORTISOL DYSREGULATION
Overarching term for abnormalities in *cortisol metabolism,* including *hypercortisolaemia.*

CORTISOL METABOLISM
The whole of chemical processes in the body involving *cortisol*.

CYTOKINE
Protein playing a role in the immune system.

DERMAL LAMELLA
Thin strip of dermis tissue formed on the outside of the hoof dermis, which plays an essential role in the adhesion of the hoof wall to the internal hoof.

DOPAMINE
Hormone and *neurotransmitter* that controls the intermediate lobe of the *pituitary gland* in the production of a group of hormones called *melanocortins*. It inhibits their production.

DOPAMINE AGONIST
A substance that resembles *dopamine* in action and therefore activates dopamine *receptors*.

DOPAMINERGIC
Responding to, releasing, or otherwise involving *dopamine*.

EMS
Equine metabolic syndrome. A cluster of interrelated metabolic problems.

ENDOCRINOPATHIC LAMINITIS
Laminitis that occurs due to hormonal issues. Therefore, also called hormone-related laminitis.

ENDOCRINOPATHY
Disease caused by the improper functioning of one or more endocrine (i.e. hormonal) glands.

ENZYME
A protein that causes, enables or accelerates a biochemical reaction.

EPIDERMAL LAMELLA
Thin strip of epidermal tissue formed on the inner side of the hoof wall, which plays an essential role in adhesion of the hoof wall to the internal hoof.

ESC
Ethanol-soluble carbohydrates. Single and double sugars, such as *glucose*, fructose and sucrose.

FREE RADICAL
Harmful molecular by-product of normal *metabolism*, inflammation, drugs, pesticides left on food, strenuous exercise, stress, *obesity* and *adiposity*.

FRUCTAN
Certain type of *WSC*.
Complex carbohydrate.

FSH
Follicle stimulating *hormone*.
Reproductive hormone.

GLUCOCORTICOIDS
A specific group of *corticosteroids*, with approximately 95% being *cortisol*. Synthetic versions of these endogenous *hormones* are also employed as drugs.

GLUCOSE
Certain type of *ESC*. Single sugar.

GLUCOSE METABOLISM
The whole of chemical processes in the body involving *glucose*.

HALF-LIFE
The time required for a quantity of a substance in the body to reduce to half of its initial value. It is an indicator of the duration of action.

HORMONE
A substance produced by various organs in the body, reaching and influencing specific organs and tissues through nerves or the bloodstream.

HYPERCORTISOLAEMIA
An elevated level of *cortisol* in the blood.

HYPERGLYCAEMIA
An elevated level of *glucose* in the blood.

HYPERINSULINAEMIA
An elevated level of *insulin* in the blood resulting from excessive insulin production and insufficient *insulin clearance*.

HYPERLEPTINAEMIA
An elevated level of leptin in the blood.

HYPERLIPIDAEMIA
Elevated levels of fats in the blood.

HYPERPLASIA
Enlargement of an organ due to abnormal cell multiplication.

HYPERTRICHOSIS
Abnormal, thick, curly and long coat resulting from a disruption of the hair growth cycle.

HYPERTRIGLYCERIDAEMIA
A form of *hyperlipidaemia* characterised by elevated levels of *triglycerides* in the blood.

HYPERTROPHY
Enlargement of an organ due to abnormal cell enlargement.

HYPO-ADIPONECTINAEMIA
A reduced level of *adiponectin* in the blood.

Hypothalamic-pituitary-adrenal axis
The system of direct (neuro)hormonal influences and feedback loops between the *hypothalamus, pituitary* and *adrenal glands*.

Hypothalamus
Part of the midbrain that lies above the *pituitary gland* and controls it.

IGF-1
Insulin-like growth factor 1. A *hormone* responsible, among other things, for the growth of cells and tissues.

Insulin
Hormone produced by the *pancreas*. It regulates *glucose metabolism*.

Insulin clearance
Breakdown and removal of *insulin* by the liver and kidneys.

Insulin dysregulation
Overarching term for abnormalities in *insulin metabolism*. In particular, *hyperinsulinaemia* and *insulin resistance*.

Insulin metabolism
The whole of chemical processes in the body involving *insulin*.

Insulin resistance
Physiological condition in which cells fail to respond to the normal actions of *insulin*.

IU/L
International units per litre. Pharmaceutical unit of measurement for a relative quantity of a substance.

Laminitis
A pathological condition in which the connection between the *dermal* and *epidermal lamellae* of the hoof becomes so damaged that the two are no longer held together. The connection between the hoof wall and the coffin bone ruptures.

Leptin
Appetite-regulating *hormone*, belonging to the *adipokines*.

Leptin dysregulation
Overarching term for abnormalities in *leptin metabolism*. In particular, *hyperleptinaemia* and *leptin resistance*.

Leptin metabolism
The whole of chemical processes in the body involving *leptin*.

Leptin resistance
Physiological condition in which cells fail to respond to the normal actions of *leptin*.

LH
Luteinising *hormone*. Reproductive hormone.

LOW-GRADE INFLAMMATION
Chronic state of inflammation of the body. The immune system is continuously active, but at such a low level that classic inflammatory signs do not occur.

MELANOCORTINS
A class of *hormones*, including *ACTH, alpha-MSH, CLIP* and *beta-endorphin*, produced by the *pituitary gland*.

MELANOTROPE
Hormone-producing cell in the intermediate lobe of the *pituitary gland*.

METABOLISM
The totality of physical and chemical processes that take place within living cells for the maintenance, breakdown and construction of tissue as well as for energy production.

MICROBIOME
Community of micro-organisms, including bacteria, unicellular organisms, yeasts, parasites, and viruses, that inhabit various parts of the body, such as the intestines.

NEURODEGENERATIVE DISORDER
Progressive deterioration of part of the nervous system.

NEUROTRANSMITTER
Endogenous chemical responsible for transmitting nerve signals.

NSAIDs
Non-steroidal anti-inflammatory drugs. Certain group of analgesic and anti-inflammatory drugs.

NSC
Non-structural carbohydrates. *WSC* and starch.

OBESITY
Type of overweight in which fat is more or less evenly distributed over the body.

OSTEOPOROSIS
Advanced stage of bone demineralisation, characterised by an increased risk of fracture.

OXIDATIVE STRESS
Cell damage due to excess oxygen bonds in a cell.

PANCREAS
Mixed gland in the duodenum that secretes *hormones*, including *insulin*, to promote the breakdown of certain nutrients.

PERGOLIDE
A substance similar to *dopamine* in its effects. It activates dopamine *receptors* in the *pituitary gland*, inhibiting the release of *melanocortins*.

PERIODONTITIS
A category of inflammatory conditions affecting the supporting tissue of the teeth.

PITUITARY GLAND
Hormone gland at the base of the brain, which secretes stimulating *hormones*. Also called hypophysis.

PITUITARY ENLARGEMENT
Enlargement of the *pituitary gland* due to *hyperplasia* and *hypertrophy*.

POMC
Pro-opiomelanocortin. A protein c.q. *pro-hormone* produced by *melanotropes* and *corticotropes*.

PPID
Pituitary Pars Intermedia Dysfunction. A *neurodegenerative disorder* of the hypothalamic *dopamine*-producing nerves that results in a loss of *dopaminergic* inhibition of the *pituitary gland's* intermediate lobe, chronic overproduction of *POMC* and its derived hormones (and an increase in their biological activity), and the development of clinical signs of the condition. *Pituitary enlargement* can lead to neurological difficulties later in the disease's course.

PRO-HORMONE
A precursor of a *hormone*. It usually has little or no hormonal effect itself.

PROLACTIN
Hormone secreted by the anterior lobe of the *pituitary gland*. The inhibition of its release is under the control of the *hypothalamus* through the action of *dopamine*.

RECEPTOR
Part of a cell, specialised in taking up (hormonal) stimuli and inducing a response under the influence of those stimuli.

REFERENCE VALUES
Two outer limits within which the results of a (blood) test are acceptable or normal.

SEASONAL RISE
Increase in *ACTH* and the derived *melanocortins alpha-MSH* and *CLIP* from mid-July to mid-November, peaking in September-October. *Beta-endorphin* probably also has this rise.

SEROTONIN
Hormone and *neurotransmitter* that affects the sleep cycle, sexual activity and appetite, among other things. It also plays a role in processing pain stimuli.

SIRS-RELATED LAMINITIS
Laminitis that occurs due to toxins in the bloodstream. Also referred to as sepsis-related laminitis.

SUBCLINICAL
Early stage of a condition, in which no recognisable or observable *clinical signs* are evident.

TRAUMATIC LAMINITIS
Laminitis that occurs due to heavy, prolonged, repetitive, or improper loading of the hooves on a hard surface. Also referred to as supporting limb laminitis or road founder.

TRH
Thyrotropin-releasing hormone. *Hormone* produced by the *hypothalamus* that triggers the *pituitary gland's* release of certain hormones.

TRIGLYCERIDE
Specific type of fat.

WSC
Water-soluble carbohydrates. ESC and fructan.

INDEX

G

garlic 109

gelding 39, 79, 81

gender 14

genetic predisposition 43

gestation 99

ginger 109

gingivitis, *see:* gum inflammation

ginkgo biloba 109

GIP 41

GLP-1 41

glucocorticoid 24, 33

glucose 85, 125

glue-on shoe 141

glutathione peroxidase 58

glycaemia, *see:* blood sugar level

glycogen 42

glycosuria 30

glyphosate 61

grain, *see:* cereal

grass 41, 52, 60, 114, 115, 116

grass pellets 119, 128

grazing 117, 121, 123

grazing muzzle 117

grazing restrictions 60

gum inflammation 36, 133

gut flora, *see:* microbiome

H

Haflinger 128

hawthorn 110

hay 41, 116, 126

hay analysis, *see:* roughage analysis

haylage 123, 127

heartbar shoe 140, 142

heat, *see:* oestrus

hemidesmosome 49, 51, 52

hepatic steatosis, *see:* fatty liver

hirsutism 30, *see also:* hypertrichosis

homeopathy 150

hoof abscess 36, 45, 50, 69, 88, 140, 142, 143

hoof (anatomy) 47

hoof boots 135, 139

hoof care provider 140

hoof mechanism 47, 140

hoof slough 135

hoof wall 49

housing 95, 104

hypercortisolaemia 21, 38, 42, 54, 102, 110

hyperglycaemia 30, 42, 51

hyperhidrosis 30, 132

hyperinsulinaemia 38, 41, 51, 52

hyperleptinaemia 38, 44

hyperlipidaemia 43, 54, 128, 150

hyperphagia 32

hyperplasia 25, 41, 54, 102

hypertension 43

hypertrichosis 28, 29, 67, 132

hypertriglyceridaemia 54, 94

hypertrophy 25, 54, 102

hypo-adiponectinaemia 44

hypohidrosis 30, 113, 132

hypophysis, *see:* pituitary gland

hypothalamic-pituitary-adrenal axis 23

hypothalamus 11, 15, 22, 23, 26, 29, 44, 58

I

IL-6 62

IL-8 36, 59

immune system 35, 62, 102, 134

immunosenescence 35

incretin 41

infection 35, 40

infertility 38, 94

inflamm-aging 35

inflammation 35, 60

influenza 60

insulin 18

insulin clearance 42

insulin dysregulation 12, 28, 30, 31, 35, 36, 38, 41, 51, 85, 124, 148

insulin metabolism 41

insulin resistance 33, 36, 41, 42, 44, 51, 52, 104, 115, 124, 128

insulin response 41, 123

insulin-response test 86

insulin test 85

intermediate lobe 15, 16, 58

internal foot 47

iron 42, 115, 118, 131, 145

K

ketoprofen 103

kidney 19

L

lab values, *see:* reference values

lamella 49, 52

lamellar connection 137

lamellar wedge 70

laminitic stance 69

laminitis 13, 28, 40, 41, 43, 45, 80, 84, 88, 94, 99, 100, 102, 103, 106, 125, 131, 135

large intestine 60, 119, 131

leptin 18, 44, 62, 85, 86

leptin and adiponectin test 86

leptin dysregulation 44

leptin resistance 32, 44

leptin test 86

levothyroxine 105

LH 38

ligament inflammation 37

ligament laxity 34

lignin 126

linseed oil 122

lipofuscin 58

liver 42

liver enzyme 72

low-grade inflammation 35, 59

lucerne, *see:* alfalfa hay

lung infection 36

luteinising hormone, *see:* LH

lysine 114, 120, 122

M

macroadenoma 26

magnesium 130, 135

manganese 145

mare 38, 79, 81, 94, 99, 110

mastitis, *see:* udder infection

meadowsweet 110

melanocortin 15, 17, 22, 28, 37, 38, 52, 92

melanotrope 16

melatonin 29

metabolite 23, 25

metformin 104

methionine 111, 114, 120, 122

microalgae 129

microbiome 119, 129

microthrombose 37

middle lobe, *see:* intermediate lobe

milk thistle 109, 110

milk yield 38, 99

mineral 114

mitochondrial dysfunction 62

MnSOD 59

monk's pepper, *see:* chasteberry

MRI 89

MSM 111

mucuna pruriens 109

mud fever 36

muesli 118

sole perforation 49, 103, 135, 145
southern hemisphere 75
soya hulls 119, 120, 122
stable rest 136
stallion 39, 81
starch 41, 80, 116, 122, 124, 125
straw 126
stress 79, 88
strip grazing 117
structural carbohydrate, *see:* SC
subclinical laminitis 33, 45, 52, 69
subclinical PPID 65, 72, 78
sucrose 125
sugar 41, 60, 116, 122, 124
sunflower oil 122
supplement 112, 129
supporting limb laminitis, *see:* traumatic
   laminitis
suprarenal gland, *see:* adrenal glands
suspensory ligament 34
suxibuzone 103
sweating, *see:* hyperhidrosis
symptom, *see:* clinical sign
synthetic shoe 143

T
tapeworm 135
teeth, *see:* dental problems
tendinitis, *see:* tendon inflammation
tendon inflammation 37
tendon laxity 34
tendon sheath inflammation 37
tendovaginitis, *see:* tendon sheath
   inflammation
tenotomy 146
testosterone 29
therapeutic shoe 141
thistle 130

3-nitrotyrosine 58
threonine 114, 120, 122
thrush 139
thyroid gland 105
thyroid hormone (synthetic) 105
thyrotropin-releasing hormone, *see:* anterior
   lobe
tissue-specific cortisol metabolism 25, 35
TNF-alpha 62
toxin 37, 40, 60
trace element 114
training 147
traumatic laminitis 49
TRH 15
TRH-stimulation test 82
triglyceride 54, 129
trilostane 102
trimming 137
tubular lobe 16
tumour 25, 26
Turkish saddle 16
turmeric 108
type 2 diabetes 104, 109

U
udder 31
udder infection 38
unbound cortisol, *see:* free cortisol
underweight 112, 121
urine 30
uterine infection 36, 38
uteritis, *see:* uterine infection
uveitis, *see:* eye infection

V
vaccination 67, 135
vasoconstriction 37, 51, 52, 53, 54, 104
vasodilation 51